THE INFLUENCE OF MATTHEW BAILLIE'S MORBID ANATOMY

BIOGRAPHY, EVALUATION AND REPRINT

Publication Number 886

AMERICAN LECTURE SERIES®

A Publication in

The BANNERSTONE DIVISION *of*
AMERICAN LECTURES IN THE HISTORY OF MEDICINE AND SCIENCE

Consulting Editor

DR. CHESTER R. BURNS

THE INFLUENCE OF MATTHEW BAILLIE'S MORBID ANATOMY

BIOGRAPHY, EVALUATION AND REPRINT

By

ALVIN E. RODIN, M.D., F.R.C.P.(C)

Professor of Pathology
University of Texas Medical Branch
Galveston, Texas

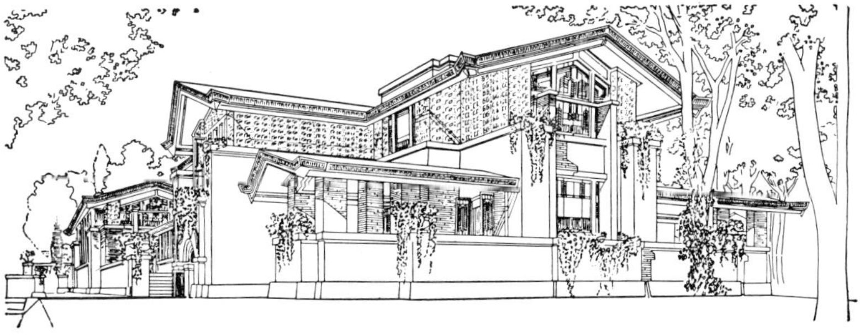

CHARLES C THOMAS • PUBLISHER

Springfield • Illinois • U.S.A.

Published and Distributed Throughout the World by

CHARLES C THOMAS • PUBLISHER
Bannerstone House
301-327 East Lawrence Avenue, Springfield, Illinois, U.S.A.

ISBN 0-398-02781-1

Library of Congress Catalog Card Number: 72-11618

With THOMAS BOOKS careful attention is given to all details of manufacturing and design. It is the Publisher's desire to present books that are satisfactory as to their physical qualities and artistic possibilities and appropriate for their particular use. THOMAS BOOKS will be true to those laws of quality that assure a good name and good will.

Printed in the United States of America
R-1

PREFACE

MATTHEW BAILLIE'S *Morbid Anatomy of the Most Important Parts of the Human Body* was one of the first pathologic works published originally in the English language, the first edition being in 1793 and its unique Atlas of engravings in 1803. The clarity, strict adherence to observation, and lack of involved discussion of suppositions was in contrast to other books of the eighteenth and nineteenth centuries. These features made it quite usable for practitioners of medicine and, as such, had an extensive influence in introducing knowledge of morphologic changes underlying clinical disease states into the daily practice of medicine. The popularity of the *Morbid Anatomy* is attested to by the need for eight English, three American and five foreign language editions.

In spite of its excellence and dependence solely on observation, unique for its time at least, Baillie's *Morbid Anatomy* has not been reprinted since 1838. Thus it is not generally available for study by students of medicine and medical history. It has not received any critical analysis in relation to other similar books of the 18th and 19th centuries, nor has its influence in establishing observation as the fundamental basis of medical knowledge been investigated.

The edition used for this reprint is the second American edition of the third London edition of 1807, which was actually a reprint of the second edition of 1797. The American editions were word for word reprints of the London ones, aside from correction of some typographical errors. The second London edition is of importance because it is the only edition of the Morbid Anatomy that had any major modification, there being a section of symptoms appended at the end of each chapter.

The reprint of the *Morbid Anatomy* in the present volume is an exact reproduction including the original variability in spelling of several words. The Table of Contents was not a feature of the original *Morbid Anatomy* but I have added it in order to provide the reader with the general layout and content of the book and to facilitate reading of selected chapters as independent units if so desired.

The primary resource material necessary for the present study was made available through the co-operation and efforts of the library staffs of the Wellcome Institute of London, the Royal College of Physicians of London, and the Royal College of Surgeons of England. Considerable assistance was provided by Ann Aldridge and Shirley Speaker in the form of typing and layout. The expert and enthusiastic guidance of Dr. Chester Burns of the Division of History of Medicine, University of Texas Medical Branch at Galveston, was instrumental in carrying out and completing this project.

A. E. RODIN

CONTENTS

		Page
	Preface	v
Matthew Baillie: Anatomist, Pathologist, Physician		3
	Introduction	5
	Biography	7
	Character	16
	The Writings of Matthew Baillie	19
	Format of Baillie's Morbid Anatomy	23
	Contributions of the Morbid Anatomy	28
	Baillie's Series of Engravings	32
Appendices		
I.	Baillie's Letter Offering his Collection	40
II.	Pathological Preparations Listed in the Catalogue of Baillie's Museum Specimens	42
III.	Papers and Autopsy Descriptions of Matthew Baillie	44
IV.	Editions and Printings of Baillie's Morbid Anatomy	47
V.	Organization and Publication of Baillie's Fascicles of Engravings of Morbid Anatomy	48
VI.	Diseases Illustrated in Baillie's Fascicles of Engravings of Morbid Anatomy	49
Reprint of Matthew Baillie's Morbid Anatomy		52
	Index	285

THE INFLUENCE OF MATTHEW BAILLIE'S MORBID ANATOMY

BIOGRAPHY, EVALUATION AND REPRINT

MATTHEW BAILLIE
ANATOMIST, PATHOLOGIST AND PHYSICIAN

INTRODUCTION

MATTHEW BAILLIE is now little known except as the last recipient of the Gold-Headed Cane, having received it from David Pitcairn's widow (1). He has not been favoured with the attention of any major biographer, there being only four relatively inaccessible eulogies published within two years after his death (2,3,4,5), a short autobiography printed in the Practitioner of 1896 (6), some notes from the diary of his wife reproduced in 1930 (7), and a brief review of his life and work in the Journal of the New Jersey Medical Society in 1961 (8).

And yet Baillie was the author of an influential book, published in 1793, that represented the first comprehensive textbook of pathology written in English. Prior to this time only Morgagni's Pathological opus of 1761 (9), Fernel's pathologic tract of 1554 (10) and Benevicni's collection of brief autopsy accounts in 1507 (11) had obtained any widespread recognition. Bichat's book on Pathology (12) was a recording of his lecture notes of 1805, transcribed by a student. It was not until Rokitansky's Pathological Anatomy of 1846 (13) that a general textbook on disease changes in the body received as widespread contemporary acknowledgment or use as Baillie's text. But Baillie remains relatively ignored in spite of the fact that his book on Morbid Anatomy went through eight English editions, three American editions and translations into Italian, French, German and Russian.

There are several reasons why Matthew Baillie has not received the attention of historians. His work in anatomy and pathological anatomy was performed under the shadow of his famous uncles, William and John Hunter. He provided little revision for succeeding editions of his textbook of Morbid Anatomy. His numerous papers relating to disease were published in journals that are now relatively obscure. Even more important is his renunciation of anatomical studies, lectures and writing at the age of 38, after which time he devoted himself completely to becoming one of the most popular private practitioners in London.

Baillie's obscurity may also be related to the nature of his textbook. It provided no hypothetical *system* of disease, as did Rokitansky's book, nor did it have any difficulties of interpretation to excite the imagination of its readers or later historians. Nonetheless it was a compact, exceptionally clear and concise account of first hand observations on disease changes. As such it was widely read and its influence on the development of disease concepts is worthy of study.

BIOGRAPHY

MATTHEW BAILLIE was indeed fortunate in the circumstances of his birth. His life span of 63 years coincided with a period of time in which Scotland and England were not disrupted by internal religious or political upheavals, although there was some social unrest due to high taxation (14). Baillie was born in 1761, only two years before the end of the Seven Years War, in which England gained control of North America and India. Baillie lived almost his entire life under one Monarch, George III, who was crowned one month before Baillie's birth and died three years before he did.

Matthew Baillie was even more fortunate in the selection of his parents. His father, the Reverend James Baillie, was more than a respected clergyman, eventually achieving the position of Professor of Divinity at the University of Glasgow. However the circumstance that influenced his life more than any other was the fact that his mother, Dorothy Baillie, was the sister of John and William Hunter, who were at the height of their anatomical and medical fame during Baillie's formative years.

The exact date of Matthew Baillie's birth was October 27, 1761. It occurred in the manse of Shotts in the County of Lanarkshire, Scotland. Soon after his birth, his father moved to the church at Bothwell and then to Hamilton. At Hamilton Baillie received his grammar school education, beginning at the age of four. At seven years of age he entered Latin School.

Baillie's university education began at Glasgow at the age of thirteen. He received a classical education in Greek and Latin as well as mathematics, logics and moral philosophy. In 1779, at the age of eighteen, he was appointed to an exhibition in Balliol College at Oxford. The nomination to these exhibitions rested entirely with the professors at the University of Glasgow, and the position of his father on the faculty may have been of some influence. However, at this time his father died, and William Hunter assumed fatherly responsibilities for him, as evidenced by Dorothy's letter to her brother:

> Dear Brother
>
> I beg leave to introduce to you my son, who is now on his way to Oxford, by London. I have furnished him out in the best manner my situation could afford. I now give him entirely to you. Be a father to him – you are the only father he has alive. I hope you shall never be ashamed of his conduct, but that he shall obey your directions in every thing. My daughters present their love to you.
>
> I am, your affectionate sister,
> Dorothy Baillie, Glasgow, March 21st, 1779, Dr. Hunter.
> Windmill Street (15).

Up to the point of Baillie's transfer to Oxford he had, to quote from his autobiographical notes, "no strong liking for this profession (medicine), as happens to some individuals, but I had no dislike for it, and entered upon it willingly" (6). A biographer of Baillie has put it somewhat more strongly – "From the peculiar advantages held out to him, by his uncle, William Hunter, he was induced, though at first contrary to his inclination, to choose medicine for his profession; at that time the pulpit or the bar would have pleased him better" (4).

In April of 1779, Baillie arrived in London and spent ten days with his uncle. He then proceeded to Oxford where he remained full-time for eighteen months, receiving additional classical education. In 1780 he returned to London to live with William Hunter and begin his medical education in earnest. His activities for the next few years were varied, and largely centered at the Hunter's Anatomical Theatre and Museum on Windmill Street. He assisted with and became quite proficient at anatomical dissection. He attended a large number of lectures – by the Hunters on surgery and dissection, by Dr. Fordyce on chemistry, the practice of physic and materia medica, and by Drs. Denman and Osborne on midwifery. Baillie was also a pupil at St. George's Hospital under John Hunter.

Baillie became a preceptual physician at the Hospital and, for one year, a Surgeon's pupil. He spent a few weeks each year at

Oxford which was only long enough "to keep up my terms."

In 1783, three years after Baillie's entrance into medical studies, William Hunter died. The terms of his will were such as one might expect if Baillie were his son. William Hunter bequeathed to him £100 per year, his anatomical theatre and house on Windmill Street and a small family estate at Long Calderwood in Scotland. Baillie in turn gave the estate to John Hunter. As part of the will the anatomy lectures were given to Baillie and Mr. Cruikshank.

Matthew Baillie bagan as an anatomy lecturer in 1782 when he was appointed teacher in the Anatomical Theatre at Windmill Street. After William Hunter's death he became a full lecturer and remained so for sixteen years. Many contemporary sources indicate that Baillie was a magnificient lecturer with a talent of making an obtruse and difficult subject plain, lucid and orderly.

> As a lecturer, he soon attained considerable eminence, being remarkable for the simplicity and perspicuity of his demonstration, the order and method of his style, and the clearness of his delivery. His manner was not without animation, yet always modest, and most unostentatious; and the attention of the student was excited, not by brilliancy, but by a remarkable fluency and precision of expression (2).

Although lecturer in anatomy, he still continued his connection with Oxford, receiving various degrees – B.A. on January 14, 1783; M.A. on June 14, 1786; M.B. on July 15, 1786; and M.D. on July 7, 1789. His medical affiliations were enhanced by appointment as Physician to St. George's Hospital on February 23, 1787, and as a Fellow of the Royal College of Physicians of London on September 30, 1789.

Baillie maintained an active role in anatomy and pathological anatomy for at least twenty years after his first association with William Hunter. Even as a practicing physician to the hospital he exhibited an intense interest in pathology. "During my situation there (St. George's) I was not only as attentive as I could be to the cases of my patients but embraced every opportunity of examining the morbid appearances after death" (6). However, his major anatomical contributions were a large collection of museum specimens and a widely used textbook of morbid anatomy.

According to the catalogue of Baillie's museum specimens, there were a total of 1281, of which almost 50 per cent were of diseased states and the remainder anatomical preparations (16). One of his early biographers (4) has credited Baillie with preparing by his own hands over nine hundred of these specimens. The remainder were preparations relating to the eye. In 1818, five years before his death, he offered the entire collection to the Royal College of Physicians, along with £400 for their upkeep (App. I). His main stipulation was that they be used primarily for the education of any Fellow Licentiate.

The collection was kept at the Royal College of Physicians until 1938, when it was offered to the Royal College of Surgeons and stored under the seats of a lecture hall until such time as it could be properly catalogued and displayed. However, during the bombing raids over London in May, 1941, the direct hit on the College building destroyed Baillie's entire museum as well as a portion of the Hunterian collection (17). All that remains is the catalogue listing the labels for each specimen (App. II). From this, Baillie's interest and industry in pathologic anatomy is evident, but it is not possible to judge his expertise.

Baillie's claim as a pathologist and as an influential personage, in the development of knowledge of disease changes, rests primarily with his textbook, *The Morbid Anatomy of Some of the Most Important Parts of the Human Body,* first published in 1793, the year of John Hunter's death (18). Its acceptance and use can be gauged by the fact that it went through eight English editions from 1793 to 1838, three American editions from 1795 to 1820 and several foreign translations – German in 1793, French in 1803, Italian in 1807, another French edition in 1815, and a Russian one in 1826.

Baillie supplemented his textbook by an illustrated atlas entitled *A Series of Engravings, Accompanied by Explanations Which are Intended to Illustrate the Morbid Anatomy of Some of the Most Important Parts of the Human Body* (19). Publication was begun in 1799, with a complete first edition in 1803 and a second edition in 1812.

Further assessment of his scientific interests can be obtained by a review of Baillie's personal library which has been housed in the library of the Royal College of Physicians of London since 1825.

There are over nine hundred volumes, mostly from the seventeenth and eighteenth centuries. All are scientific works except for a biography of John Hunter by Adams. Most are related to specific diseases such as venereal, cancer, yellow fever, rickets, inflammation and smallpox. There are a surprising number of works on pharmacology, chemistry, physiology and physics. Morgagni's work on pathologic anatomy is included. In general the library is indicative of a pragmatic and scientifically oriented physician.

We are indebted to James Wardrop for collecting Baillie's various journal and other publications in *The Works of Matthew Baillie, M.D., Vol. I,* published in 1825 (4). Under *Miscellaneous Papers* there are twenty-four contributions, all related to morbid appearances of disease (App. III). Another section is headed *Dissections* and consists of thirty-nine short autopsy descriptions of various cases, some of which describe related symptoms. Unfortunately, these contributions are not all dated, but appear to have been written before 1799.

The year 1799 was a major turning point in the professional activities of Matthew Baillie. He dropped all activities to devote full time to the private practice of medicine, giving up not only his appointment to St. George's Hospital, but also relinquishing his lectures in anatomy at Windmill Street. Baillie's reasons for dropping his lectures can be given in his own words. "I contrived as a lecturer in anatomy for fifteen years, but as my connection with W. Cruikshank, who had a very odd temper, became more and more unpleasant to me, and as my business as a physician began coincidentally to increase, I gave up altogether my situation as an Anatomical Teacher in the year 1799" (6).

Baillie's activities as a practicing physician began with his appointment to St. George's Hospital in 1787. Apparently he began private practice at about this time, at first not too successfully. By his own account his income from practice was £100 per year in 1791 and £500 to £600 in 1795 (6). By 1797, in part because Dr. Pitcairn had relinquished his extensive practice to him, Baillie was sufficiently well established to be working sixteen hours a day.

Wardrop summarized Baillie's abilities as a practitioner by saying that "His comprehensive knowledge of anatomy, therefore, could not fail to give him immense advantages over those who were competing with him for private practice. Dr. Baillie possessed, in an eminent degree, a facility in distinguishing diseases" (3). Baillie himself, though, was somewhat more modest – "I know better perhaps than another man, from my knowledge of anatomy, how to discover a disease, but when I have done so, I don't know better how to cure it" (4).

Some insight into Baillie's method of practice is given by MacMichael (1) – "He appeared to lay a great stress upon the information which he might derive from the external examination of his patient, and to be much influenced in the formation of his opinion of the nature of the complaint by this practice." But then MacMichael criticizes this method because there may be "great disordered action" which may not be "sensibly felt," and because "one of the inevitable consequences of such a system is frequent disappointment in foretelling the issue of the malady."

After his transformation from anatomist to full time practitioner in 1799, Baillie rapidly became one of the most renowned physicians in London. He was made a member of the Royal Societies of London and England. He served as president of the Royal Society of Medicine in 1808, and was the first President of the Medical Chirurgical Society. His prominence is evidenced by his appointment as one of the physicians for Princess Amelia, the youngest child of George III, in 1810. After her death within a year, he became physician to Princess Charlotte and His Majesty's Physician Extraordinary.

Baillie was also a successful practitioner from a monetary point of view. He amassed a fortune large enough to have a town house in Lower Grosvenor Street and a country estate at Duntisbourne, and to leave his widow £1,000 a year and each of two sisters an annuity of £150 (7).

Baillie was reputed to be one of feeble physical frame, slender form and under the middle stature (Plate 1). However, he was not handicapped by serious illness until his terminal episode. In 1823 he became seriously ill with cough, fever, tracheitis, anorexia, emaciation and a pulse over 100. He was bothered by swelling of the left foot and hand and intermittent confusion of intellect (7). Although his sickness was attributed by some to overwork, Charles

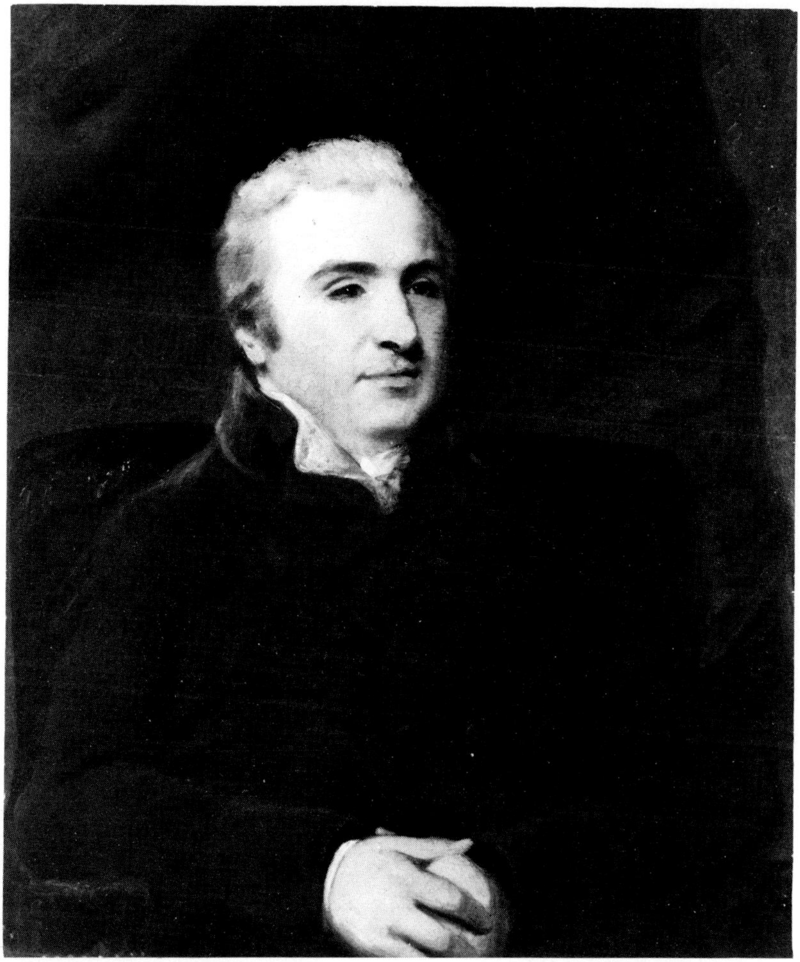

Plate 1. Matthew Baillie, circa age 40, oils on canvas, 30 by 25 inches, by John Hoppner, Courtesy of Royal College of Physicians of London.

Bell (2) suspected "some local source of irritation or visceral affectation which was preying on his constitution."

Matthew Baillie died on September 23rd, 1823, and was buried at his country home at Duntisbourne in Gloucestershire. His reputation was such that his medical friends raised sufficient money by subscription for a monument in St. James Chapel in Westminster Abbey. It consists of a bust of Baillie by Sir Francis Chantrey. Similar busts are displayed at both the Royal College of Physicians and the Royal College of Surgeons in London (Plate 2).

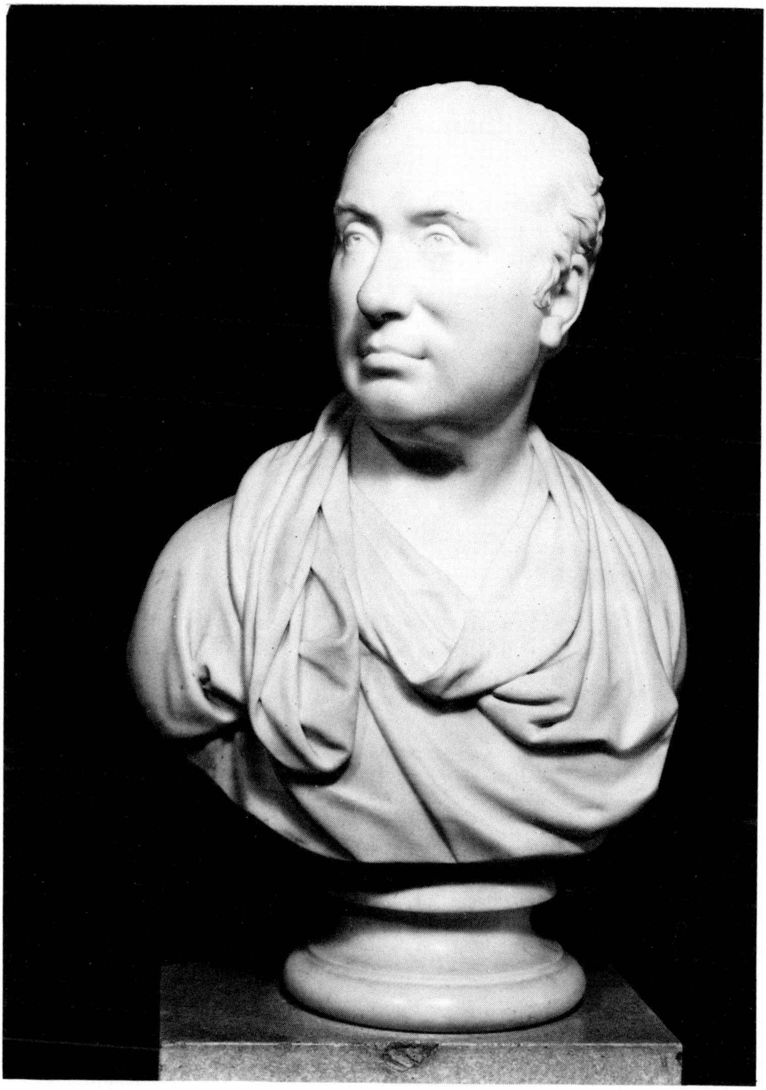

Plate 2. Matthew Baillie, circa age 50, marble bust, by Joseph Nollekens, Courtesy of Royal College of Surgeons of England.

CHARACTER

AN assessment of Baillie's character at this distant time is difficult. His earlier eulogizers may be excused some overstatement – "For Modesty, for Justice, for Fidelity, for a sacred regard to Truth, where shall we find Dr. Baillie's equal? As a Teacher, as an Author, as a Physician, and as a Man, when shall we see his like again?" (2).

There is evidence that he could be quite generous. On receipt from Laennec in 1819 of two copies of his book on auscultation, Baillie replied with a most laudatory letter (20). Wardrop records that he often refused to take fees and that on one occasion gave an impoverished tubercular patient sufficient money to spend the winter in a milder climate (4). Another example of Baillie's generosity was his contribution, in conjunction with Sir Everard Home, of £1,684 to the Royal College of Surgeons for the establishment of an annual Hunterian Oration (21).

Nonetheless, Baillie was not universally regarded with esteem by all. The fourth edition of Roberton's work on the generative system contains a particularly scathing denunciation of Baillie (22). Roberton had obtained permission to dedicate the first edition of his work to Baillie. But then Baillie objected on the basis that it was critical of Sir Everard Home's works on stricture of the urethra, Home being a relative of Baillie's by marriage of his sister to John Hunter. He also denounced it as an obscene work of indecent nature. Perhaps it was for that age, dealing with Lues Venerea arising from sexual intercourse and containing anatomical plates of the male and female genitalia.

That Baillie had some strength of character may be indicated by his association in the anatomy lecture series for sixteen years with Cruikshank, reputed to have been of a difficult nature (4). Wardrop (4) has commented that Baillie frequently became irritable with the pressure of practice, but had sufficient insight to resist arguments at these times with his wife, Dr. Denman's daughter whom he had married in 1791.

Some degree of modesty is indicated by his refusal to be created a Baronet. However, he did accept the offer to become an Honorary Fellow of the Royal College of Physicians of Edinburgh.

A perusal of Baillie's brief autobiography (6) leaves the impression of a relatively formal, self-pretentious and self-righteous individual of somewhat forced modesty. However, this orientation and style of writing about one's self may have been characteristic of his period.

A critical appraisal of Matthew Baillie can be found in MacMichael's *The Gold-Headed Cane,* first published in 1827, four years after his death (1). In fact one receives the impression that the *cane* did not fully approve of Baillie – "My present was the very reverse, in almost every particular, of my early master, Dr. Radcliffe. In person Dr. Baillie was considerably below the middle size, with a countenance rather plain than prepossessing, a Scotch dialect, and blunt manners." Furthermore, "he was sometimes rather irritable, and betrayed a want of temper in hearing the tiresome details of an unimportant story."

The *cane's* orientation towards Baillie's private practice was even more cynical. "Dr. Baillie acquired business early by the credit of his book on Morbid Anatomy. From the date of its first publication in 1793, its materials must have been furnished principally by a careful inspection of the diseased preparations collected in the museum of his uncle, Dr. Hunter."

It is apparent that Matthew Baillie had characteristics that would have brought him to eminence in any field of endeavour. He was hard-working, dedicated and had the ability to organize his activities and writings in an extremely clear and concise manner. His abrupt abdication from anatomical studies and writings is reminiscent of Vesalius's renunciation (23). There are also interesting similarities between William Osler and Matthew Baillie (24). Both had a strong orientation to pathological anatomy during their medical training and early years of practice. Both prepared many museum specimens of diseased organs and wrote many papers related to pathologic anatomy. Baillie, as Osler, was an expert diagnostician for his time and had considerable concern for his patients. And finally, both Osler and Baillie gave up pathological anatomical activities to become full time clinicians, Baillie rather abruptly and Osler more gradually.

THE WRITINGS OF MATTHEW BAILLIE

IF Baillie's book on Morbid Anatomy has received little historical recognition, his other publications have been virtually ignored. The journals in which he published are now relatively obscure or have ceased to exist many years ago. Thus one of the few descriptions of absence of the pericardium was in the *Transactions for the Improvement of Medical and Chirurgical Knowledge* of 1793 (25), and a detailed account of transposition of viscera in *Philosophical Transactions* of 1788 (26).

We are indebted to James Wardrop who collected Baillie's publications and published them in two volumes in 1825 (4), only two years after Baillie's death. Wardrop was born in 1872, by coincidence in the Scottish Parish adjoining Baillie's birthplace. His medical studies encompassed Paris, Vienna, London and Edinburgh (27). Wardrop began medical practice in Edinburgh in 1804 and then moved to London in 1809. He became Surgeon-extraordinary to the Prince Regent and was a member of the College of Surgeons.

The first volume of Wardrop's collection contains a biography of Baillie and reprints of Baillie's *Miscellaneous Papers* and *Dissections* (App. III). The *Dissections* are very brief descriptions of autopsies, somewhat similar in format to Benevieni's collection of the early sixteenth century (11). Unfortunately references to the original journals of publication are not given and only some are dated. Some, at least, were first presented before the Royal Society of Surgeons (26). The second volume consists of a revised re-issue of Baillie's *Morbid Anatomy.* The items included in *Miscellaneous Papers* are also discussed in Baillie's textbook but in a much abbreviated form. Therefore a study of the papers provides a clearer and more detailed insight into the orientation and influence of Baillie.

Baillie's *Papers* are distinguished by their precise and logical arrangement and sequence. For example, *Paraplegia in Adults* (28) begins with a definition, presents current theories, gives his own theory, describes an autopsy case and finally discusses various treatments and their rationale. Baillie's orientation is clearly that of observation. He does not consider paraplegia to be caused by disease in the bones or ligaments of the spine for the simple reason that he has seldom found this, except rarely for tumors. Although his own experience led him to postulate that the disease exists most commonly in both hemispheres of the brain, he cautioned that "The morbid appearances in this disease have not been sufficiently investigated by dissection." Baillie's experience with paraplegia may have been less extensive than that of Morgagni who previously had described a case due to severance of the spinal cord by a knife wound of the neck (29).

Baillie's discourse *On Want of a Pericardium in the Human Body* (25), follows the same pattern but provides a more detailed account of autopsy findings and of possible clinical-pathological correlations. The anatomical description includes not only the lack of the parietal pericardium but also the minute details of the relationship of the *naked* heart to the pleura, pulmonary veins, phrenic nerves, diaphragm and sternum. In contradistinction, Morgagni, in reviewing the same anomaly, denied its existence and attributed all such cases to adhesions of the pericardium (30).

Baillie was quite conversant with the medical literature of his own and previous times. He referred to seven previous reports of absence of the pericardium. A recent review of pericardial deficiencies (31) has listed eight case descriptions prior to Baillie's publication, but only two of these references are in common. Congenital defects of the pericardium are not mentioned by Bichat (12), and are by Rokitansky (32) but with no reference to clinical implications.

Baillie's concern with clinical-pathological correlations is well illustrated by his publication on pericardial absence (25). He denied that the large heart in his patient was due to the absent pericardium, on the basis that it does not normally constrain the heart because they grow together. Ellis et al (31) in 1959 indicated that 50 per cent of cases have enlarged hearts, but that in most instances the enlargement is due to "more prosaic cardiac disease." Baillie and Ellis et al, separated by 166 years of phenomenal growth in medical knowledge, both doubt any function of the pericardium in respect to heart position, the former because other structures keep the heart in place, and both because individuals with pericardial absence often have a normal life span and no related symptoms. The only additional concept in the 20th century is that the pericardium may protect the heart from pleural infection.

Baillie was concerned not only with clinical-pathological correlations but also with pathogenesis, as exemplified by his paper on diabetes (33). After presenting an autopsied case, he discussed at length the various theories in existence. He rejected the concept that diabetes is due to a morbid state of the liver, such as steatomatous collections, because many diabetics have normal livers. Also unlikely is retrograde flow of chyle from lacteals into kidney lymphatics because such anastomoses have not been demonstrated and because chyle is not very sweet. Also diabetes is not likely due to escape of chyle into relaxed urinary tubules because, if they were relaxed, *red globules* should also escape into urine, and this is not seen. This analysis by Baillie is indicative of a rejection of suppositions and a reliance on logic based upon direct observation.

Baillie went even further in applying observation to test hypotheses. He killed two dogs, one that had been on a normal diet and one fed only bread and butter (33). Chyle from the former was not sweet and from the latter was only slightly sweet – again contrary to the chyle hypothesis of diabetes. This is one of the first recorded animal experimentations on diabetes, Minowski's dog pancreatectomies not being performed until 1889 (34). Unlike Baillie, Morgagni's account of diabetes is quite rambling and unprecise (35). In the next century, Rokitansky's opus on pathology did not even index diabetes (13).

Baillie's papers are remarkable for his time in that they were not concerned with any *system* of disease causation. However his strong inclination to observation did not preclude him from making some generalizations regarding etiology. For example in his paper on situs inversus totalis (26), there is a comprehensive discussion of congenital malformations in general and of the possible basis for their deviation from the norm. He concluded that "it is exactly the same creative action which produced the natural structure, or any deviation from it; for in cases of deviation the action is either carried too far, ceases too soon, or is diverted into uncommon channels. This will explain the various kinds of monstrosity from redundancy, deficiency or transposition of parts." Such a concise and logical statement is in considerable contrast to the writings of Morgagni in 1761 (36) and Rokitansky in 1845 (37), both of whom placed much emphasis on the effect of maternal emotions on the development of specific malformations.

Baillie's paper on situs inversus (26), one of the first such descriptions, also provides evidence for an extensive experience with many detailed autopsy dissections. He was quite familiar with anatomical variations, such as bone markings and blood vessel distribution, and that these variations do not interfere with function. He was sufficiently experienced to realize that there is little normal variation in the nervous system and organs of sense. In these publications one can appreciate the wealth of observation and the clarity of thought that served as the foundation for Baillie's Morbid Anatomy.

FORMAT OF BAILLIE'S MORBID ANATOMY

MATTHEW BAILLIE published *The Morbid Anatomy of Some of the Most Important Parts of the Human Body* (18) at the age of thirty-two, ten years after assumption of the lectures in anatomy on William Hunter's death and six years before his abdication to the full-time practice of medicine. The book appeared thirty-two years after Morgagni's De sedibus (9) and forty-nine years before Rokitansky's Pathologische Anatomie (13). This period of eighty-one years was characterized by numerous descriptions of pathologic states such as intussusception by John Hunter, congenital pyloric stenosis by Armstrong, spinal caries by Pott, peritonitis by Laennec, meningitis by Vusseux, appendicitis by Parkinson, scleroderma by Alibert, lymphadenoma by Hodgkin, and nephritis by Bright (38). However there was only one book on pathological anatomy, other than Baillie's, published originally in English, Clossy's *Observations on Some of the Diseases of the Parts of the Human Body* (39).

Clossy's book had limited exposure because there was only one *small edition,* unlike Baillie's Morbid Anatomy which reached eight editions. It has recently been rescued from oblivion by Saffron who produced a facsimile reprint in 1967 (40). Samuel Clossy received his M.B. from Trinity College of Dublin in 1751 and his M.D. in 1756. He delivered Lectures in Anatomy at King's College Medical School and performed autopsies at Stevens Hospital. In 1763, at the time of his immigration to New York, he published privately in London his slender volume of observations on diseases. Baillie was only two years old at the time and, because of the limited edition, may well have not encountered it during his anatomical and medical studies.

Clossy's text is organized on the basis of fifty-three case reports, each with a short history including a brief autopsy description, and followed by a lengthy discussion of various hypotheses. It resembles, in fact, a miniature of Morgagni's De Sedibus (9) which was published two years earlier. Baillie's Morbid Anatomy, however, had a completely different format, not being dependent on specific cases, but being structured according to each system and the various disease changes that can occur therein. The only case history in the entire book is that of a young man with an abscess of the pancreas. Indeed the format of the Morbid Anatomy is similar to that used by Fernel in his brief pathologic treatise (10), published 239 years previously.

Baillie's Morbid Anatomy consists of twenty-four chapters, beginning with the pericardium and ending with the brain. The first edition of 1793 (18) is dedicated to Sir George Baker President, and the Fellows of the Royal College of Physicians of London, the professional organization to which Baillie was most devoted. The preface includes a very succinct rationale for writing the book. "The object of this work is to explain more minutely than has hitherto been done, the changes of structure arising from morbid actions in some of the most important parts of the human body." Baillie certainly succeeded in overcoming some of the detrimental features of Morgagni's opus which he lists as too general descriptions, too much detail of "smaller collateral circumstances" and too large for general use by practitioners.

The preface to Baillie's Morbid Anatomy also contains justifications for an intimate knowledge of morbid anatomy, each of which could well be re-emphasized for our modern chemical and molecular age in which the autopsy has been greatly depreciated: – foundation for determining morbid actions, distinguish between erroneous theories, lead to better treatment and more accurate diagnosis, and acquire a "knowledge of the whole disease." One of the major attributes of Baillie's work may well be that it placed more emphasis on direct observation than on hypothesis.

A comparison of the eight editions of the Morbid Anatomy reveal relatively few changes from the original. The second edition of 1797 received more alterations and additions than any succeeding edition. The dedication was now changed to Dr. David Pitcairn who had relinquished much of his practice to Baillie, and whose widow was to give him the gold-headed cane (1). A major addition was an account of symptoms at the end of each chapter. Although his discussion of clinical-pathological correlations may be rather primitive for our modern tastes, the generalities given in the preface to the second edition are particulary incisive and astute for the seventeenth century. For example, some symptoms may be associated with different morbid changes, some morbid changes may have different symptoms, patients may explain imperfectly their feelings, morbid changes may have no corresponding symptoms and, especially, medical men may ask inaccurate and misleading questions. Such comments are indicative of a wide experience and careful study of clinical histories and related autopsy findings.

Numerous changes for the second edition of the Morbid Anatomy were written by Baillie in an interleaved copy of the first edition (41), now located in the library of the Royal College of Physicians of London. Nonetheless the changes consisted only of added or altered phrases and sentences. For example, he added that bony conversion of the pericardium is "very uncommon," that the larynx may have a violent catarrh as does the trachea, that disease spread to the trachea would produce difficulty in breathing, that he has never seen an ulcer starting on the outer surface of the intestine and spreading, that piles are dilatation of veins and not arteries as claimed by some anatomists, that scirrhous of the liver is not like scirrhous elsewhere, that ulcers of the cervix are not unusual, and that a dead fetus in the uterus can be converted into an earthy mass. Also added to the second edition was the first mention in print of "rheumatism of the heart."

Other additions in the second edition (42) included ossification of the coronary arteries, aneurysm of the internal carotid artery, accumulation of water in the substance of the lung, air vesicles attached to the edge of the lung, diseases of the thymus and a description of several worms such as taenia and trichinosis. He now discussed an opening in the diaphragm through which the intestine enters the thorax. He considered its cause to be bursting or malformation of the diaphragm, and made the critical observation that it impedes the functions of the circulation and respiration so that newborns die almost immediately after birth.

Evidently many of the changes in the second edition were instigated by Professor Soemmerring of Germany who translated the first edition into German and sent Baillie a detailed critique. The Professor's suggestions are alluded to relatively frequently but not always with agreement. For example Baillie retained his statements that coagulated lymph is alive even though Soemmerring was not satisfied with the proof, and that black colored gallstones are not soluble in water in spite of the Professor's experience.

The third edition of the Morbid Anatomy in 1807 (43) can be dispensed with briefly for reasons given by Baillie in its Advertisement. He was not able to make any additions as "for the past seven years I have been so much engaged in the practical duties of my profession." The same can be said for the fourth edition of 1812 (44) which was in essence a reprint. The Advertisement to the fifth edition of 1818 (45) stated that it was somewhat enlarged with the help of notes from the 1807 Italian and 1815 French editions. However changes are not readily apparent.

It is problematical whether or not to consider the 1825 issue of *The Works of Matthew Baillie, M.D., Vol. II* by James Wardrop (4) as the sixth edition because Wardrop made his own major imprint on the work. He added lengthy "preliminary observations on diseased structures" and many topics in the chapters. Wardrop's observations can be categorized as general pathology with comments on abnormal growth and destruction by diseases, primary (main site) and secondary (elsewhere) stages of diseases, scrofula, ultimate *contamination* of lymphatic glands by most cancers, etc. Some of the additional topics introduced by Wardrop include air in the pericardium, excrescences of the heart valves, melanoid tubercles of the lung, warts on the larynx, and diseases of the omentum. Although some of these additions were quite useful, they did not alter the basic nature of Baillie's Morbid Anatomy.

A seventh issue of the Morbid Anatomy occurred in 1830 (46). Although called a *new edition* it was in effect a reprint of the 1818 fifth edition. The eight and last edition was published in 1838 (47) and was a reprint in a small, pocket-sized format. Thus Baillie's Morbid Anatomy had an active period of publication for almost half a century, from 1793 to 1838, lasting for fifteen years beyond his demise in 1823.

All English editions of Baillie's text were published in London (App. IV), the first five by Johnson and Nicol. Wardrop's sixth edition was published by Longman, Hurst, Rees, Orme, Brown and Green with the qualification "to which are prefixed preliminary observations on diseased structures by the editor." The seventh edition was called *a new edition* and published by E. Limebeer. The eighth edition was so labelled by the publishers Cox and Portwine.

The foreign editions are of considerable interest because they provide evidence that Baillie's Morbid Anatomy had a widespread influence. Each of the three American issues were published at different places – Albany, Walpole and Philadelphia. The German publication was translated by Dr. Soemmerring, Professor of Medicine at the University of Mayence, who added "many new Cases and Copious Notes." However, the French edition, translated by Dr. Ferrall, was a direct translation with no additions. Similarly the Italian translation by Dr. Pietro Gentilini, was a faithful rendition of the second edition.

Less well known, and indicative of a still broader influence of the Morbid Anatomy, is the existence of a Russian translation of 1826, described by J. A. Shilinis of Moscow at the International Congress of the History of Medicine in London, September, 1972. Baillie's text was translated by Ivan Kostomarov, professor of the Moscow Medico-Surgical Academy. He added "his own Treatise on the relation of morbid anatomy to other medical sciences, as well as on methods with the help of which it may be cognizable and perfected." His comments included a plea to "comprehend changes in vital function" which accompany morbid changes. This Russian translation, along with the other foreign editions, extended familiarity with and use of Baillie's Morbid Anatomy to three continents, Asia, Europe and North America.

CONTRIBUTIONS OF THE MORBID ANATOMY

THE numerous reprints of Baillie's Morbid Anatomy are indicative that it fulfilled a real need in the first part of the nineteenth century. According to Esmond Long (48) "in spite of all its solid achievements, the seventeenth century failed to attain a working codification of this knowledge (pathologic anatomy). Indeed this was finally reached in a form useful to physicians only in the closing years of the eighteenth century in the text and atlas of Matthew Baillie." However his statement, that "This book is the first text of pathology devoted to the science (pathology) exclusively by systematic arrangement and design," overlooks Fernel's pioneering book (10) over two centuries previously.

Not only the brevity of the Morbid Anatomy but also the clearness and conciseness of the language contributed to its popularity. Baillie had the gift of not only being able to lecture effectively but also to write superbly. Another factor in the widespread acceptance of the Morbid Anatomy may have been its freedom from long dissertations of hypothetical mechanisms of etiology and pathogenesis. Unlike Morgagni's work (9), in which morphologic descriptions of disease are buried within massive rambling discussions, Baillie's book was largely limited to naked eye appearances. Thus it effectively highlighted and popularized knowledge of the morphologic basis of diseases.

The Morbid Anatomy contains several specific *firsts.* The most striking of these is Baillie's description of cirrhosis, under the designations of common tubercle of the liver and scirrhus liver. The description of the cirrhotic liver is quite detailed, including small and large types of tubercles, increased firmness and decreased size. In contrast, Morgagni's huge work (9) and Clossy's minor book (39) do not specifically mention this entity, and

Rokitansky's description (13) forty-nine years later adds nothing. Garrison (49) has given Baillie credit for the first accurate definition of cirrhosis.

More intriguing is the suggestion that Baillie was the first to relate cirrhosis of the liver to alcoholism (50,51). "This disease is hardly met with in a very young person, but it is likewise more common in men than in women. This seems to depend upon the habit of drinking being more common in one sex than in the other; for this disease is more frequently found in hard drinkers" (18). Baillie's avoidance of unfounded theorizing is apparent in the following statement where he stated simply that, although no connection is apparent between cirrhosis and alcoholism, "very commonly we can see little connection between cause and effect."

Credit for the first delineation of an association between cirrhosis and alcoholism has also been given to William Heberden (52). In his Commentaries of 1802 (53), he makes a statement on cirrhosis almost identical to that of Baillie who, in fact, preceded him by nine years. The source of Heberden's insight is not apparent, but in the case of Baillie the correlation is indicative of astute clinical and morphologic observation.

Baillie has also been credited with the first gross delineation of another major disease, emphysema (54). His description, titled "Air Cells of the Lung enlarged," is brief but terse. "The lungs are sometimes, although I believe, rarely formed into pretty large cells, so as to resemble somewhat the lungs of an amphibian animal. Of this I have now seen three instances." His gross description preceded Laennec's classic clinical presentation of emphysema (55) by thirty-seven years. However Baillie did, in his section on symptoms, relate emphysema to patients "long subject to difficulty of breathing."

Rokitansky (13), who provided the first microscopic description, gives credit to Laennec for the first delineation of emphysema. However, even before Baillie, Morgagni (56) described an autopsy in which "The cavity of the thorax was almost wholly fill'd by the lungs, being very turgid, and heavy; but still less heavy than turgid; for they contain'd a great quantity of air, and not much serum; for which reason they were soft, and of natural color." Nonetheless it was Baillie who first referred to the basic abnormality of dilated alveoli. According to Major (57), the lungs described by Baillie belonged to Samuel Johnson.

Although Baillie was not prone to any lengthy theorizing he did include a few comments on the development of emphysema. "The enlargement of the cells cannot well be supposed to arise from any other cause, than the air being not allowed the common free egress from the lungs, and therefore accumulating in them. It is not improbable also, that this accumulation may sometimes break down two or three continguous cells into one, and thereby form a cell of a very large size" (18). No basically new concept of the pathogenesis of chronic obstructive emphysema has been added in the succeeding 150 years. However Baillie did not relate "air vesicles attached to the side of the lungs" to emphysema because they did not appear to communicate with underlying air cells.

Although priority of recorded observations is most clearly apparent in Baillie's references to cirrhosis and emphysema, many of his descriptions of clinical-pathologic relationships and pathogenesis, if not the first, were quite sophisticated for his time. Examples include formation of peritoneal and pleural adhesions by inflammation, absorption of hemorrhage in the brain leaving cavities, hydatids arising from retained placenta, pain in the right shoulder resulting from inflammation of the liver, atrophy of one optic nerve in unilateral blindness, relation of ascites to cirrhosis and large spleen, and distention of vena azygos due to obstruction of the inferior vena cava. The clarity and conciseness of these statements in the widely published Morbid Anatomy undoubtedly popularized the concept of diseases having observable cause and effect relationships.

Baillie was quite aware of recent advances in medical science as indicated by his statement that angina pectoris is related to coronary ossification. The first clear recording of this relationship was by Parry in 1799 (58), at about the time Baillie added it to his second edition (and gave proper credit for it). Baillie also provided clear statements of pathogenesis of morphologic changes. For example "Aneurysms at the arch of the aorta, as well as in every other part of the arterial system, arise from the coats of the artery being previously diseased, which are thereby unable to resist sufficiently the impetus of blood that strikes against them. This is obvious, both from the diseased structure of the coats of an aneurysm itself, and of the artery in its neighbourhood." In such a manner does Baillie clear away the stiffling suppositions of the middle ages and lay the basis for a more realistic appraisal of disease processes.

Baillie was in the vanguard of the *scientific* approach to medicine of the nineteenth century in several other ways. He provided not only detailed descriptions of gallstones and urinary calculi but also results of chemical analyses of these structures. He was familiar with functional reserve of the kidney and compensatory renal hypertrophy. Baillie was quite aware of the fact that post-mortem changes occurred in organs such as the brain and stomach, and that polypi of the heart represented only coagulation of blood after death.

The main strength of the Morbid Anatomy, however, lies in the careful and accurate descriptions of diseased changes, uncluttered by excess wordage or unfounded supposition. His descriptions of worms provide exquisitely minute details. His account, of "little white spots being formed in the inner membrane of the artery (arch of aorta), and its coats being more easily separable from each other than in the healthy state," is quite recognizable as syphilitic aortitis.

These concise statements, on which Baillie's Morbid Anatomy was based, were made on his own autopsies and on specimens in the Hunterian museum, for which he gives ample credit (as, for example, in references to ruptured heart valve and malformed hearts). But the value of his book also lies in the fact that he was a practicing clinician and made as astute observations on patients as he did on their organs. It was this combination of experience in both anatomy and medical practice, in an individual gifted with clarity of vision, thought and statement, that resulted in the first practical and useful textbook of pathology and clinical pathologic relationships.

BAILLIE'S SERIES OF ENGRAVINGS

BAILLIE'S Morbid Anatomy was complemented by *A Series of Engraving Accompanied with Explanations, which are Intended to Illustrate the Morbid Anatomy of Some of the Most Important Parts of the Human Body* (19). Surprisingly, the first of these engravings were published at about the time of Baillie's abdication from the study of anatomy and disease to the full-time practice of medicine in 1799. His justification for their publication, as given in the first fascicle, was "No work has been published in this, nor, I believe, in any other country, in which the principle Morbid Changes of Structures, affecting the most important parts of the Human Body, have, as far as they admit of it, been illustrated by a Series of Engravings" (19). And, indeed, Krumbhaar has given him credit for the first such Atlas (59).

Baillie's series of engravings were published as ten separate fascicles from December 8, 1798 to October 30, 1802, and collated as a first edition in 1803 (19). The dedication, as for the second and succeeding editions of the Morbid Anatomy, was to David Pitcairn. There are ten fascicles, each consisting of from six to nine plates with each plate followed by a description (App. V). Because each plate contains from two to five figures, there are a total of eighty-one diseases represented in the engravings (App. VI). Orientation to the figures are enhanced by labeling with letters. The sequence in the Series of Engravings corresponds to that of the Morbid Anatomy.

Baillie gave full credit for contributions to his Series of Engravings. For each figure the source of the specimen used is given, mostly from his own preparations and those in Dr. Hunter's museum. The drawings were done by *a young Man,* Mr. William Clift (later to become Conservator of the Royal College of Surgeons). The plates were prepared by engravings on steel of his drawings.

Unlike the Morbid Anatomy, the Series of Engravings saw only a second edition, nine years after the first, in 1812. The contents are identical to the first but the layout somewhat inferior. The index of the first edition was not included and descriptions of all plates in each fascicle were placed together before the plates.

The caliber of the Series of Engravings must be seen to be appreciated. The drawings themselves are as clear and concise as their accompanying descriptions and as those in the Morbid Anatomy. For example, the figure of emphysema (Plate 3) was sufficiently striking to be reproduced by Major in his *Classic Descriptions of Disease* (57). Enlarged alveoli of variable size are clearly represented and referred to as "shewing a large cellular structure." The figure beside it is diagnosed as ossified lung, and may represent an old tubercular lung.

Another superb drawing is that of cirrhosis (Plate 4). It effectively highlights the large and variable-sized nodules on both the capsular and cut surfaces, so much so that the figure can readily be labeled today as post-necrotic scarring of the liver. The plate of figures on heart valve disease is also quite explicit (Plate 5). Figure 5-1, demonstrating short thick aortic cusps, are more likely rheumatic than leutic because of the absence of widening of the commissures. Figure 5-3, a calcific aortic stenosis, provides an excellent graphic illustration of valvular rigidity.

These are only a few examples from Baillie's Series of Engravings. Taken in its totality, the atlas is a remarkable achievement for the beginning of the nineteenth century. When placed in context with his Morbid Anatomy, it provides sufficient justification for calling Baillie the first modern descriptive pathologist.

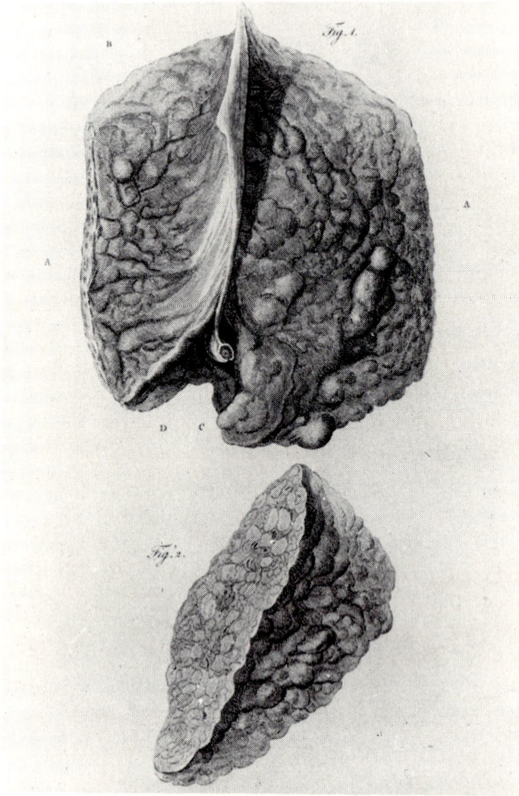

Plate 3. In this Plate are exhibited two very rare diseased appearances of the lungs, the one an enlargement of their cells, and the other an ossification of their substance. From Matthew Baillie's Series of Engravings (19), Fascicle Two, Plate VI.

Figure 3-1. Represents a section of one of the lungs, exhibiting the first kind of disease. In this section the air-cells are seen much enlarged beyond their natural size, so as to resemble the air-cells of the lungs in amphibious animals.

A. The external surface of this section of the lungs.

B. Its cut edge, shewing a large cellular structure. The very dark cavities, which are about ten in number, are the orifices of some divided branches of the pulmonary blood vessels and the trachea.

From the Author's Collection.

Figure 3-2. Represents lungs which had been ossified to a great extent.

A. The trachea.

BB. The two bronchia.

CCCCC. The ossified portions of the lungs.

The parts which appear of a dark colour, consist of the natural substance of the lungs dried. The lungs are here represented as being considerably smaller than the natural size; but this was necessary, in order that they might be adapted to the size of the Plate.

From Mr. Hunter's Museum.

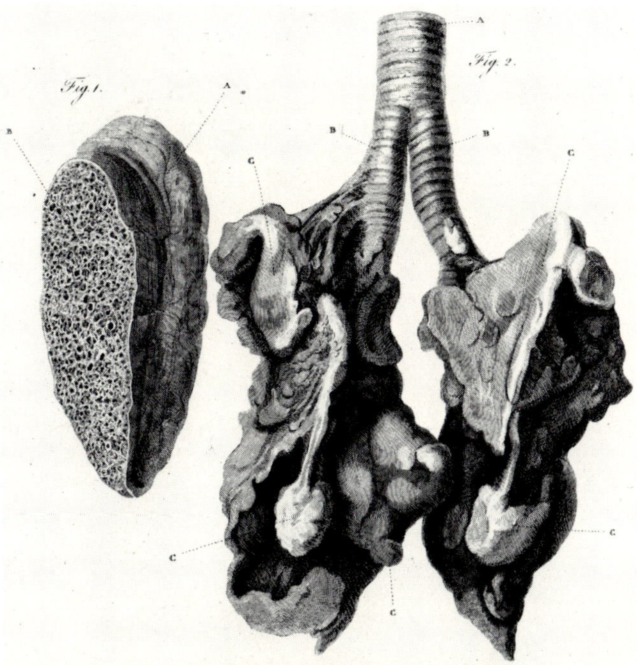

Plate 4. This Plate is intended to illustrate the most common kind of tubercle formed in the liver. The process by which they are formed is very slow, although it varies in this respect a good deal in different individuals, and it is commonly produced by a long habit of drinking spirituous liquors. When the liver has undergone this change, it is commonly said to be scirrhous, but the morbid appearance is very different from what is observed in the genuine scirrhus of other glands. It should rather be considered as a disease *sui generis*. From Matthew Baillie's Series of Engravings (19), Fascicle Five, Plate II.

Figure 4-1. Represents a considerable portion of the liver studded with tubercles.

AA. A part of the anterior surface of the liver, rendered very uneven from the irregular elevation of the tubercles.

B. A part of the suspensory ligament of the liver.

C. A section of the ligamentum terest, which, before birth, constituted a part of the umbilical vein. Although it has got the name of ligament, yet it does not change into a true ligamentous substance, but retains very much the original structure of a vein, the cavity only being obliterated.

D. The lower end of the deep fissure which separates the right and left lobe of the liver from each other.

From Mr. Heaviside's Museum.

Figure 4-2. Represents a smaller section of the liver affected with the same disease. It is intended to shew that the tubercles are not merely formed near the surface of the liver, but throughout the whole of its substance as may be distinctly perceived through the whole extent of its cut edge. In the cut edge may also be seen a few found cavities, which are sections of veins. The liver in this disease is not enlarged in its size, but is, on the contrary, somewhat diminished.

From the Author's Collection.

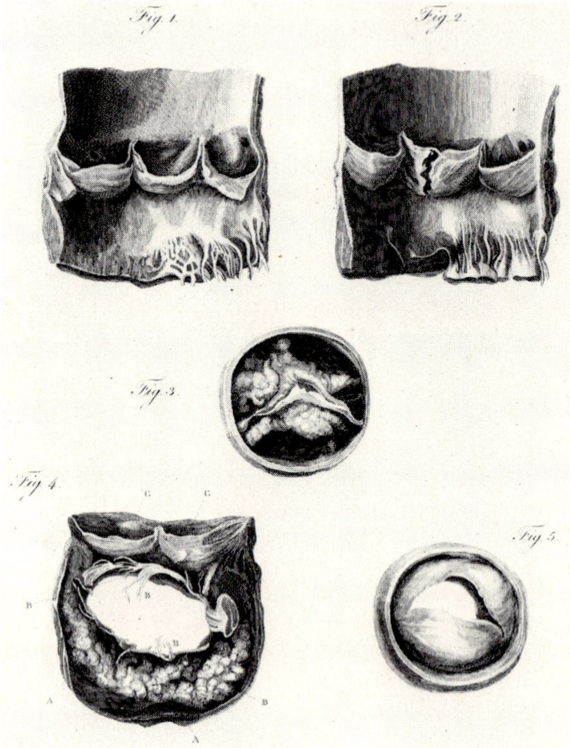

Plate 5. This Plate is intended to illustrate the diseased alterations of structure, to which the valves of the heart are subject. These consist chiefly in the valves becoming thick and opaque, or becoming ossified. The valves at the origin of the aorta are more liable to be affected with both kinds of disease, than those at the beginning of the pulmonary artery, and are more particularly subject to ossification, than the valves between the auricles and the ventricle. From Matthew Baillie's Series of Engravings (19), Fascicle One, Plate II.

Figure 5-1. Shews the three semilunar valves at the origin of the aorta, shortened in their depth, and considerably thickened. It is obvious that such valves must perform their office imperfectly.

From Mr. Hunter's Museum.

Figure 5-2. Shews one of the valves at the origin of the aorta thickened and ruptured. The other two valves are in their natural state.

From Dr. Hunter's Museum.

Figure 5-3. Shews the semilunar valves at the origin of the aorta, much ossified. The separation between two of the valves is in a great measure obliterated.

From Mr. Hunter's Museum.

REFERENCES

1. MacMichael, W.: The Gold-Headed Cane. Springfield, Thomas, 1953.
2. Bell, C.: Biographical Notice of the Late Doctor Baillie delivered by Mr. Charles Bell to the students of Anatomy and Surgery, in Great Windmill Street on the first meeting of the winter session of 1823. Reprinted and Presented to Them as the Example of a Professional Life. Wellcome Institute History of Medicine Library, 43509.
3. Wardrop, J.: Biographical Sketch of the Late Matthew Baillie, M.D. Reprinted from Edinburgh Medical & Surgical Journal, Jan. 1824, Vol. 21, Wellcome Institute History of Medicine Library, Biographical Pamphlets, No. 18a (5).
4. Wardrop, J.: The Works of Matthew Baillie, M.D. to which is Prefixed an Account of His Life collected from Authentic Sources. In 2 vols., Longman, Hurst, Rees, Orme, Brown and Green Pub., Paternoster Row, 1825.
5. Duncan, A.: Testimony of Veneration for the Memory of Dr. Matthew Baillie of London. Read at the Forty-fourth Anniversary Festival of the Harveian Society of Edinburgh, on the 12th of April, 1825. London, Longman, 1825.
6. Bailey, J. B.: Heroes of Medicine. Matthew Baillie. An Autobiography. Entitled "A Short Memoir of my Life, with a View of Furnishing Authentic Materials." Practitioner, 57:51-65, 1896 (original hand-written copy in Library of Royal College of Surgeons of England. A hand-copied version by Baillie's son is in the Library of the Royal College of Physicians of London).
7. Peachey, G. C.: Matthew Baillie, M.D. The Med Press & Circular, 180:472-474, 1930.
8. Henderson, A. R.: Matthew Baillie 1761-1823. Author of the First Comprehensive Text and Atlas of Morbid Anatomy. J Med Soc New Jersey, 58:606-611, 1961.
9. Morgagni, G. B.: The Seats and Causes of Diseases Investigated by Anatomy. Trans. by B. Alexander of 1761 ed., 1769 (Facsimile ed., 3 vols., New York, Hafner, 1960).
10. Sherrington, C.: The Endeavour of Jean Fernel. Cambridge, Cambridge U. Press, 1946.
11. Benevieni, A.: The Hidden Causes of Disease. Trans. by C. Singer from the 1507 ed., Springfield, Thomas, 1954.
12. Bichat, X.: Pathological Anatomy. The Last Course. Recorded by P. A.

Beclard in 1805, Trans. by J. Tongo, Jon Grigg, Philadelphia, 1827.
13. Rikitansky, C.: A Manual of Pathological Anatomy. Trans. by W. E. Swaine of 1846 ed., 4 vols., London, Sydenham Society, 1854.
14. Woodward, E. L.: A History of England. London, Methuen, 1962.
15. Wardrop (4), p. xiii.
16. Baillie, M.: Catalogue of Anatomical and Pathological Preperations in the Museum of the Royal College of Physicians, London. London, Hunterian Museum, Royal College of Surgeons of England, undated mss.
17. Dobson, J., personal communication, 1971.
18. Baillie, M.: The Morbid Anatomy of Some of the Most Important Parts of the Human Body. 1st ed., London, Johnson and Nicol, 1793, 314 pp.
19. Baillie, M.: A Series of Engravings, Accompanied by Explanations, which are Intended to Illustrate the Morbid Anatomy of Some of the Most Important Parts of the Human Body. 1st ed., London, Johnson and Nicol, 1803, 288 pp. 73 plates.
20. Le Fanu, W. R.: Laennec and Matthew Baillie. Ann Royal Coll Surg, 36:67-68, 1965.
21. Kobler, J.: The Reluctant Surgeon: A Biography of John Hunter. Garden City, Doubleday, 1960, p. 320.
22. Roberton, J.: On The Generative System: Fourth Edition to which are prefixed Letters by Matthew Baillie, M.D. London, Stockdale, 1817.
23. O'Malley, C. D.: Andreas Vesalius of Brussels. Berkeley, U. of Calif. Press, 1964.
24. Rodin, A. E.: Canada's Foremost Pathologist of the Nineteenth Century. William Osler. Canad Med Assoc J, 1972.
25. Baillie, M.: On the Want of a Pericardium in the Human Body. Trans Soc for the Improvement of Med & Chirurg Knowledge, 1:91-101, 1793.
26. Baillie, M.: An Account of a Remarkable Transposition of the Viscera. Philosoph Transact, 78(2):350-363, 1788.
27. Hill, B.: A Pioneer in Surgery, James Wardrop, M.D., F.R.C.S., 1782-1869. The Practitioner, 202:302-306, 1969.
28. Wardrop (4) Paraplegia in Adults, Vol. I, Misc. Papers, pp. 1-8.
29. Morgagni (9) Vol III, Letter LIII, Article 23, pp. 184-185.
30. Morgagni (9) Vol I, Letter XXIII, Article 17, pp. 695-696.
31. Ellis, K.; Leeds, N. E., and Himmelstein, A.: Congenital Deficiencies in the Parietal Pericardium. Amer J Roentgen, 82:125-137, 1959.
32. Rokitansky (13) p. 131.
33. Wardrop (4) An Account of a Case of Diabetes with an Examination of the Appearances after Death, pp. 94-111.
34. Wrenshall, G. A.; Hetenyi Jr., G., and Feasby, W. R.: The Story of Insulin. Toronto, Reinhardt, 1962, p. 44.
35. Morgagni (9) Vol II, Letter XLI, Article 15, pp. 462-463.
36. Morgagni (9) Vol II, Letter XLVII, Article 54, pp. 758-760.
37. Rokitansky (13) Vol I, p. 11.
38. Garrison, F. H.: An Introduction to the History of Medicine. Phila-

delphia, Saunders, 1929, Appendix I, 996 pp.
39. Clossy, S.: Observations on Some of the Diseases of the Parts of the Human Body. Chiefly Taken from the Dissections of Morbid Bodies. London, Kearsley, 1763, 196 pp.
40. Saffron, M. H.: Samuel Clossy, M.D. (1724-1786). The Existing Works with a Biographical Sketch. New York, Hafner, 1967.
41. Baillie, M.: The Morbid Anatomy of Some of the Most Important Parts of the Human Body. Interleaved copy, 1st ed., 1793, Royal College of Physicians of London.
42. Baillie, M.: The Morbid Anatomy of Some of the Most Important Parts of the Human Body. 2nd ed., London, Johnson and Nicol, 1797, 460 pp.
43. Baillie, M.: The Morbid Anatomy of Some of the Most Important Parts of the Human Body. 3rd ed., London, Johnson and Nicol, 1807, 461 pp.
44. Baillie, M.: The Morbid Anatomy of Some of the Most Important Parts of the Human Body. 4th ed., London, Johnson and Nicol, 1812, 470 pp.
45. Baillie, M.: The Morbid Anatomy of Some of the Most Important Parts of the Human Body. 5th ed., London, Cox and Sons & G. and W. Nicol, 1818, 482 pp.
46. Baillie, M.: The Morbid Anatomy of Some of the Most Important Parts of the Human Body. A new ed., London, Limebeer, 1830, 248 pp.
47. Baillie, M.: The Morbid Anatomy of Some of the Most Important Parts of the Human Body. 8th ed., London, Cox and Portwine, 1838, 281 pp.
48. Long, E. R.: A History of Pathology. New York, Dover Pub., 1965.
49. Garrison, F. H.: An Introduction to the History of Medicine. Philadelphia, Saunders, 1929.
50. Galambos, J. T.: Alcohol and Liver Disease. Am J Digest Dis, 14:477-486, 1969.
51. Paton, A.: Liver Disease. Philadelphia, Lippincott, 1970.
52. Secretary Health, Education and Welfare: Alcohol and Health. U.S. Dept. Health, Education and Welfare, December, 1971, p. 47.
53. Heberden, W.: Commentaries on the History and Cure of Diseases. London, Payne, 1802.
54. Larson, R. K.: Historical Note on Emphysema. Am Rev. Resp Dis, 91:277-278, 1965.
55. Laennec, R. T. H.: A Treatise on the Diseases of the Chest and on Mediate Auscultation. Trans. by John Forbes. New York, Wood and Sons, 1830.
56. Ref. 9, Letter IV, Article 24.
57. Major, R. H.: Classic Descriptions of Disease. 3rd ed., Springfield, Thomas, 1945.
58. Parry, C. H.: An Inquiry into the Symptoms and Causes of the Syncope Anginosa, commonly called Angina Pectoris: Illustrated by Dissection. Bath., 1799.
59. Krumbhaar, E. B.: Clio Medica. Pathology. Reprint edition. New York, Hafner, 1962.

APPENDIX I

BAILLIE'S LETTER OFFERING HIS COLLECTION*

My Dear Sir,

I think it proper to communicate to you in writing the substance of the Conversation which we had together at your house last night.

I propose to give in the course of this season my Anatomical Collection to the President and Fellows of the Royal College of Physicians in London, and their successors forever. This collection contains above a thousand Preparations in Bottles, by far the greater number of which was made by my own hands. In order that the College may be at no expense in preserving the Collection in good condition, I propose to give at the same time to the College, Four Hundred Pounds Sterling, the interest of which I know from long experience will be an ample fund for this purpose. The four hundred Pounds should, I think, be laid out in Stock, either the Consols or any other of Government, which the College may think adviseable.

I wish the Collection to be open for three hours in the Forenoon during two days of each week, *not for shew,* but to give an opportunity to any Fellow or Licentiate to examine any Preparations which may be useful to them in their Researches. By extending this permission to the Licentiates, the Collection will be render'd much more useful to the Public.

The Preparation or Preparations should be examined in the room where the Collection is placed, and should not be carried out of the College. Some Gentleman appointed by the College should be in the Room where the Collection is, the whole of the three

---

*Original on file at the Royal College of Physicians of London.

hours, that it is open as above-mentioned.

You are all at liberty to communicate the Contents of this Letter to the College when ever for please.

I remain, my dear Sir,
Yours very faithfully
(signed W. Baillie)

Lower Grosvenor Street
October 8, 1818
To Dr. Latham President

P.S. If you will be so good as call in Lower Grosvenor Street on Thursday morning next at half past Nine oclock, I shall show you the bulk of the Collection, by which you will be enabled to judge better about a Room in the College fitted to receive it.

APPENDIX II

PATHOLOGICAL PREPARATIONS LISTED IN THE CATALOGUE OF BAILLIE'S MUSEUM SPECIMENS*

Organs of Motion	No. of Specimens
Morbid Anatomy of the Bones	18
Organs of Digestion	
Morbid Anatomy of the Gullet	6
Morbid Anatomy of the Stomach	8
Morbid Anatomy of the Intestines	80
Hernia	9
Morbid Secretions from the Bowels	9
Intestinal Worms	33
Anatomy & Morbid Anatomy of the Liver	36
Hydatids of the Liver	5
Morbid Anatomy of the Spleen	6
Morbid Anatomy of the Absorbents	5
Organs of Circulation and Respiration	
Morbid Anatomy of the Heart and its Vessels	36
Aneurisms	17
Morbid Anatomy of the Larynx, Trachea & Lungs	44
Secretions Expectorated	3
Urinary Organs	
Morbid Anatomy of the Kidneys	31
Morbid Anatomy of the Bladder	11

*Original in Hunterian Museum of the Royal College of Surgeons of England (16).

Organs of the Senses	No. of Specimens
Morbid Anatomy of the Brain and Nerves	51
Morbid Anatomy of the Organs of Smelling	3
Morbid Anatomy of the Organ of Sight	2
Morbid Anatomy of the Organ of Feeling	11
Organs of Generation	
Morbid Anatomy of the Male Organs	20
Morbid Anatomy of the Uterus	26
Morbid Anatomy of the Ovaries	34
Monstrous Productions, Malformations	6

Note: The number of specimens is listed on 6 index cards within the Catalogue. The total number is 1281 of which 39 per cent are related to diseased organs or tissues. In 1938, 1251 specimens were transferred from the Royal College of Physicians of London to the Royal College of Surgeons of England.

APPENDIX III

PAPERS AND AUTOPSY DESCRIPTIONS OF MATTHEW BAILLIE*

Miscellaneous Papers

Observations on Paraplegia in Adults
Additional Observations on Paraplegia
Case of Hydrocephalus with Separation of the Bones of the Cranium
Case of Internal Hydrocephalus with uncommon Symptoms
Observations on a strong Pulsation of the Aorta in the Epigastric Region
Uncommon Appearances of Disease in Blood Vessels
Obliteration of Blood Vessels
Ossification of Blood Vessels
The Want of a Pericardium
Cases of Inflammation of the Mucous Membrane of the Larynx and Trachea
Emphysema, not proceeding from Local Injury
Remarkable Hardness of the Skin of an Infant
An Account of several Persons who had the Measles twice
Additional Instances of the same
Observations respecting the Green Jaundice
Case of Diabetes and Appearances after Death
Case of a Man who had no Evacuation from the Bowels for nearly fifteen weeks before death
Separation and Discharge of a Portion of the Great Intestine
Stricture of the Rectum produced by Spasmodic Contraction
Observations respecting a particular Species of Purging

*Collected by James Wardrop in "The Works of Matthew Baillie, M.D., Vol. I," published by Longman in 1825 (4).

A particular Change of the Structure in the Ovarium
Remarkable Transposition of the Viscera
Remarkable Deviation from the Natural Structure in the Urinary Bladder
On Embalming Dead Bodies

Dissections

Regeneration of the Rete Mucosum
Case of Locked Jaw
Destruction of a Portion of the Mucous Coat of the Stomach
Case of Ulceration of the Stomach
Mucus of the Stomach
Malformation of the Liver
Rupture of the Liver
Tubercles of the Liver
Scrophulous Abscesses in the Liver
Conversion of the Vesiculae Seminales into a fatty Substance
Division of the Urinary Bladder into Two Chambers
Fungus of the Bladder
Urinary Fistula
Scrophulous Tumours on the Peritoneum and Mesentery
Universal Adhesion of the Abdominal Viscera
State of the Intestines from fatal Purging
Contents of the Intestinal Canal at Birth
Ulcers of the Mucous Membrane of the Gall Bladder
Inflammation of the Larynx
Enlargement of the Vena Cava
Obliteration of the Right Carotid Artery
Aneurism of the Aorta
Scrophulous Tubercles of the Lungs
Effusion of Air into the Cellular Membrane of the Lungs
Case of Peritoneal Inflammation, produced by the Escape of Urine into the Cavity of the Abdomen
Interitis mistaken for Colic
Tumor of the Thoracic Duct
Extra-uterine Conception
Dissection of an Impregnated Uterus

Muscular Structure of the Uterus
Ovarium containing Fat and Hair
Singular Disease of the Muscles
Ossification of the Internal Intercostal Muscle
Singular Disease of a Nerve
Bone formed in different Organs
Diseased Appearances in Typhus Fever
Fungus Haematodes of the Arm
Malformation of the External Ear

APPENDIX IV

EDITION'S AND PRINTINGS OF BAILLIE'S MORBID ANATOMY

English

First Edition (18)	1793	London	314 pp.
Second Edition (42)	1797	London	460 pp.—numerous minor changes additions of symptom sections
Third Edition (43)	1807	London	461 pp.—reprint of 2nd edtition
Fourth Edition (44)	1812	London	470 pp.—reprint of 2nd edition
Fifth Edition (45)	1818	London	482 pp.—some minor additions
Wardrop Edition (4)	1825	London	—preliminary observations and additional topics by Wardrop
A New Edition (46)	1830	London	248 pp.—same as fifth edition
Eighth Edition (47)	1838	London	281 pp.—same as fifth edition

American

First Edition	1795	Albany	248 pp.—from 1st edition
Second Edition	1808	Walpole	271 pp.—from 3rd edition
Third Edition	1820	Philadelphia	288 pp.—from 5th edition

French

First Edition	1803
Second Edition	1815

German

First Edition	1794

Italian

First Edition	1815

Russian

First Edition	1826

APPENDIX V

ORGANIZATION AND PUBLICATION OF BAILLIE'S FASCICLES OF ENGRAVINGS OR MORBID ANATOMY (19)

Number	*System*		*Published*
Fascicle I	Heart	6 plates	Dec. 8, 179
Fascicle II	Lungs, Thyroid, Larynx, Trachea, Pleura	6 plates	June 24, 179
Fascicle III	Pharynx, Esophagus, Stomach	7 plates	Jan. 25, 180
Fascicle IV	Intestine	9 plates	June 20, 180
Fascicle V	Liver, Pancreas	7 plates	Nov. 1, 180
Fascicle VI	Spleen, Kidney	8 plates	March 1, 180
Fascicle VII	Urinary Bladder	6 plates	July 20, 180
Fascicle VIII	Seminal Vesicles, Prostate, Urethra, Testicles	8 plates	Dec. 1, 180
Fascicle IX	Female Organs	8 plates	Apr. 20, 180
Fascicle X	Cranium, Brain, Membranes	8 plates	Oct. 30, 180

APPENDIX VI

DISEASES ILLUSTRATED IN BAILLIE'S FASCICLES OF ENGRAVINGS OF MORBID ANATOMY (19)

Pericarditis
Valvular Disease
Aneurysm Aorta
Calcific Pericarditis
Monstrosity of Heart (Transposition of Great Vessels)*
Enlargement of Thyroid (Goiter)
Abscess of Thyroid
Croup of Trachea (Diphtheria)
Calcified Pleura
Pleurisy
Abscess of Lung
Tubercles of Lung
Tubercles of Lung (Metastatic Tumors)
Enlarged Air Cells of Lung (Emphysema)
Foreign Body in Esophagus
Thrush
Tumors of Esophagus
Ulcers of Esophagus
Stricture of Esophagus
Ulcers of Stomach
Cancer of Stomach
Stricture of Stomach
Scrofula of Intestines (Tuberculosis)
Peritonitis
Adhesions of Peritoneum

---

*Note: In parenthesis – diagnostic interpretation by A. E. Rodin, M.D.

Dysentery
Cancer of Rectum
Fistulae in Ano
Piles (Hemorrhoids)
Rectum Imperforated (Anus)
Polyp of Colon
Stricture of Intestine
Inguinal Hernia
Diaphragmatic Hernia
Intestinal Worms
Abscess of Liver
Tubercles of Liver (Cirrhosis)
Hydatids of Liver
Gall Stones
Obstruction Bile Duct
Chronic Pancreatitis
Calculi Pancreatic Duct
Abscess Spleen
Tubercles of Spleen
Splenomegaly
Abscess Kidney
Renal Stones
Hydatids of Kidney (Cysts)
Scrofula of Kidney (Tuberculosis)
Hypertrophy of Bladder
Ulcer of Bladder
Calculi of Bladder
Diverticuli of Bladder
Polyps of Bladder
Tumor of Bladder
Scrofula of Seminal Vesicles (Tuberculosis)
Calculi of Prostate
Abscess of Prostate
Scirrhus Prostate (Hyperplasia)
Stricture of Urethra
Perineal Fistulae
Hydrocele
Inflammation of Testicle

Cancer of Uterus
Tumor of Uterus (Leiomyoma)
Scirrhus Uterus (Hypertrophy)
Polyps of Uterus
Prolapsed Uterus
Inversion of Uterus
Cyst of Ovary
(Dermoid Cyst of Ovary)
Hydatids of Tube (Hydatidiform Mole)
Bony Tumors of Cranium
Venereal Disease of Cranium
Hydrocephalus
Inflammation of Membranes (Leptomeningitis)
Ossification Dura Matter
Tumor of Dura Matter
Abscess of Brain
Tubercles of Choroid Plexus
Hemorrhage of Brain

THE
MORBID ANATOMY
OF SOME
OF THE MOST IMPORTANT PARTS
OF THE
HUMAN BODY

By

MATTHEW BAILLIE, M.D.F.R.S.

FELLOW OF THE ROYAL SOCIETIES OF LONDON AND
EDINBURGH, AND FELLOW OF THE ROYAL
COLLEGE OF PHYSICIANS IN LONDON

THE SECOND AMERICAN
FROM THE THIRD LONDON EDITION
CORRECTED

WALPOLE: N.H.

PRINTED BY G. W. NICHOLS
FOR W. FESSENDEN, BOOKSELLER
DRATTLEBOROUGH, VT.

. . . .

1808

CONTENTS

Of the Morbid Anatomy*

PREFACE TO THE FIRST EDITION 67

PREFACE TO THE SECOND EDITION 71

ADVERTISEMENT TO THE THIRD EDITION 74

CHAPTER I–DISEASED APPEARANCES OF THE PERICARDIUM 75

Inflammation of the Pericardium 75
Adhesions of the Pericardium to the Heart 77
Dropsy of the Pericardium 78
Scrofulous Tumours in the Pericardium 79
The Pericardium almost dry 79
The Pericardium cartilaginous, and bony 80
The Pericardium wanting 80
SYMPTOMS 81

CHAPTER II–DISEASED APPEARANCES OF THE HEART 83

Inflammation of the Heart 83
White Spot upon the Surface of the Heart 83
Polypus 84
Aneurysm of the Heart 85
Aneurysm of the Arch of the Aorta 86
Ossification of the Coronary Arteries of the Heart 88
Ossification of the Semi-lunar Valves 88
Semi-lunar Valves thick and opaque 88

*Compiled by A. E. Rodin

Rupture of the Valves 88
Valves between the Auricles and the Ventricles ossified . . 88
The same Valves thick and opaque 89
Rupture of the Heart 89
Blood in the Pericardium, without a Rupture of the Heart 89
Malformation of the Heart 90
Heart enlarged 92
Hydatids adhering to the Heart 92
A Portion of the Heart bony, or earthy 93
SYMPTOMS 93

CHAPTER III–DISEASED APPEARANCES IN THE CAVITY OF THE THORAX 96

Inflammation 96
Adhesions in the Cavity of the Thorax 97
Empyema 97
Hydrothorax 98
The Pleura almost dry 99
Ossification of the Pleura 99
SYMPTOMS 100

CHAPTER IV–DISEASED APPEARANCES OF THE LUNGS 103

Inflammation 103
Abscesses 104
Tubercles 105
Soft pulpy Tubercle 106
Water accumulated in the substance of the lungs 107
Lungs distended with Air 107
Air Cells of the Lungs enlarged 107
Air Vesicles attached to the Edge of the Lungs 108
Lungs changed into a substance like Liver 108
Lungs converted into Bone 108
A solid Tumour compressing the Lungs 109
Earthy Concretions in the Lungs 109

Hydatids 109
SYMPTOMS 110

CHAPTER V–DISEASED APPEARANCES OF THE THYROID GLAND, THE LARYNX, AND THE PARTS CONTAINED IN THE POSTERIOR MEDIASTINUM 112

Inflammation of the Thyroid Gland 112
Bronchocele 112
Scirrhous of the Thyroid Gland 113
The Thyroid Gland converted into Bone 114
Larynx–The cartilages of the Larynx converted into Bone 114
Ulcers in the cavity of the Larynx 115
Diseased Appearances of the Parts contained in the Posterior Mediastinum 115
Diseased Appearances of the Trachea 115
Appearances of the Trachea in the Croup 116
Polypus 116
Trachea scirrhous 117
Rings of the Trachea ossified 117
Ulcers of the Trachea 118
Diseased Appearances of the Oesophagus 118
Spasmodic stricture of the Oesophagus 118
Stricture from the puckering of the inner Membrane of the Oesophagus 119
Stricture attended with Ulcer 119
Oesophagus cartilaginous 120
Fungus in the Pharynx 120
Scrofulous swelling in the Pharynx 121
Pouch formed at the lower end of the Pharynx 121
The descending Aorta 122
The Vena Azygos varicose 122
Vena Azygos ruptured 122
The Thoracic duct varicose 123
Thoracic Duct obstructed 123
Thoracic Duct ruptured 123

Absorbent Glands scrofulous 123
Absorbent Glands scirrhous 124
Absorbent Glands bony 124
The Anterior Mediastinum 124
Diseased Appearances of the Thymus Gland 125
SYMPTOMS 125

CHAPTER VI–DISEASED APPEARANCES WITHIN THE CAVITY OF THE ABDOMEN 130

Ascites 130
Inflammation of the Peritonaeum 131
Adhesions in the Cavity of the Abdomen 132
Scrofulous Masses adhering to the Peritonaeum 133
Cancerous Tumours adhering to the Peritonaeum 134
Cartilaginous Excrescences growing from the Peritonaeum 134
Steatomatous Tumours adhering to the Peritonaeum . . . 134
Hydatids in the Abdomen 134
Air in the Cavity of the Abdomen 135
SYMPTOMS 135

CHAPTER VII–DISEASED APPEARANCES OF THE STOMACH 138

Inflammation 138
Appearances in the Hydrophobia 139
Ulcers of the Stomach 139
Scirrhous and Cancer of the Stomach 140
Circumscribed scirrhous Tumours in the Stomach 141
Pouch formed in the Stomach 141
Stricture at the Pylorus 141
Stomach much contracted, or much enlarged 142
Stomach distended with Air 142
Part of the Stomach dissolved by the Gastric Juice 143
Fatty Tumours in the Stomach 143
Calculi in the Stomach 144
Morbid Papillae observed in the Stomach 144

Small-pox Pustules said to be in the Stomach 144
SYMPTOMS 144

CHAPTER VIII–DISEASED APPEARANCES IN THE INTESTINES 146

Inflammation 146
Intus-Susceptio 149
Ruptures 149
Hernia Congenita 152
Scirrhus and Cancer of the Intestines 153
The diseased Change of the intestines in Dysentery 154
Thickened Folds of the Inner Membrane of the Great Intestines 155
Piles 155
Fistulae in Ano 156
The Rectum terminating in a Cul-de-sac 156
The Rectum terminating in the Bladder 157
Worms 157
Lumbricus Teres 157
Taenia 159
Taenia Solium 159
Taenia Lata 160
Ascaris 161
Trichuris 161
Air accumulated in the Intestines 161
Bony Matter formed in the Intestines 162
Projecting Ring formed in the Cavity of Jejunum 163
Calculous Matter in the Intestines 163
Small-pox Pustules said to be in the Intestines 163
Diseased Appearances of the Mesentery –Mesentery Inflamed 163
Mesenteric Glands scrofulous 164
Mesenteric Glands cancerous 164
Mesenteric Glands earthy or bony 164
SYMPTOMS 165

CHAPTER IX–DISEASED APPEARANCES OF THE LIVER 169

Inflammation of the Membrane of the Liver 169

Adhesions 169
Coats of the Liver converted into Cartilage 170
Inflammation of the Substance of the Liver 170
Common Tubercle of the Liver 171
Large White Tubercle of the Liver 172
Soft brown Tubercles of the Liver 173
Scrofulous Tubercles of the Liver 173
Liver flaccid, with reddish Tumours 174
Liver very soft in its Substance 174
Liver very hard in its Substance 174
Hydatids 175
Cysts in the Liver containing an Earthy Matter 177
Rupture of the Liver 177
Worms said to be in the Liver 178
SYMPTOMS 178

CHAPTER X–DISEASED APPEARANCES IN THE GALL-BLADDER 181

Inflammation of Its Coats 181
Adhesions 181
Ulcers in the Gall-Bladder 181
Coats of the Gall-bladder thickened, and hard Tubercles formed in them 182
Coats of the Gall-bladder bony 182
Diseased state of the Biliary Ducts. –Their Dilatation 182
Obliteration of the Biliary Ducts 183
A preternatural Canal of Communication between the Gall-bladder and the Stomach 183
Gall-stones 183
Bile 186
Gall-Bladder distended with Bile 186
Hydatids in the Gall-bladder 186
The Gall-bladder wanting 186
SYMPTOMS 186

CHAPTER XI–DISEASED APPEARANCES OF THE SPLEEN 189

Inflammation of the Coats of the Spleen 189

Adhesions 189
Inflammation of the Substance of the Spleen 189
The Spleen extremely soft 190
The Spleen very hard 190
Tubercles in the Spleen 191
Coats of the Spleen Cartilaginous 191
Spleen very large 191
Hydatids in the Spleen 192
Stony Concretions in the Spleen 192
The Spleen ruptured 192
Several small Spleens 192
Spleen said to be wanting 193
SYMPTOMS 193

CHAPTER XII–DISEASED APPEARANCES OF THE PANCREAS 195

Abscess of the Pancreas 195
Pancreas hard 195
Calculi of the Pancreas 195
Pancreas wanting 196
SYMPTOMS 196

CHAPTER XIII–DISEASED APPEARANCES OF THE KIDNEYS AND THE RENAL CAPSULES 198

Capsules of the Kidneys inflamed 198
Abscesses of the Kidneys 198
Scrofulous Tubercles in the Kidneys 199
Kidney Scirrhus 199
State of the Kidneys in Diabetes 199
Kidneys very soft 200
Hydatids of the Kidneys 201
Calculi of the Kidneys 202
Kidneys earthy and bony 203
Original Varieties in the Kidneys 203
Diseased Appearances of the Renal Capsules 204
Abscess in the Renal Capsules 204
Renal Capsule scrofulous 204
SYMPTOMS 205

CHAPTER XIV–DISEASED APPEARANCES OF THE BLADDER 207

Inflammation of the Peritonaeal Covering 207
Inflammation of the Inner Membrane 207
Ulcers 208
Scirrhus and Cancer 209
Fungous Excrescences 209
Polypus of the Bladder 209
Elongation of the inner Membrane 210
Cysts communicating with the Bladder 210
Muscular Coat Thickened 210
The Bladder divided into two Chambers 212
Calculi 213
Bladder Distended 216
Bladder Contracted 216
The anterior part of the Bladder wanting 216
The Bladder and the Rectum communicating from original Malformation 217
Part of the Bladder in a hernial Sack 217
SYMPTOMS 217

CHAPTER XV–DISEASED APPEARANCES OF THE VESICULAE SEMINALES 220

Vesiculae Seminales inflamed 220
Vesiculae Seminales scrofulous 220
Ducts of the Vesiculae Seminales terminating in a Cul-de-sac 221
Vesiculae Seminales very small 221
One of the Vesiculae Seminales wanting 221
Vesiculae Seminales scirrhous 221
SYMPTOMS 222

CHAPTER XVI–DISEASED APPEARANCES OF THE PROSTATE GLAND 223

Abscess in the Prostate Gland 223
Scrofula of the Prostate Gland 223
Scirrhus of the Prostate Gland 223

Calculi in the Ducts of the Prostate Gland 225
Ducts of the Prostate Gland enlarged 225
The Prostate Gland preternaturally small 225
SYMPTOMS 226

CHAPTER XVII–DISEASED APPEARANCES OF THE URETHRA 227

Abscesses 227
Fistulae 227
Stone in the Cavity of the membranous part of the Urethra 227
Cowper's Glands seldom observed to be diseased 228
Inner Membrane of the Urethra inflamed 228
Ulcers in the Urethra 229
Stricture 229
Caruncle 229
A layer of earthy matter in the urethra 230
Preternatural Orifice of the Urethra 230
SYMPTOMS 230

CHAPTER XVIII–DISEASED APPEARANCES OF THE TESTICLES, AND THE SPERMATIC CHORD 232

Hydrocele 232
Hydatids 233
Loose Cartilages in the Tunica Vaginalis Testis 233
Adhesions 233
Testicle inflamed 233
Abscesses of the Testicle 234
Testicle scrofulous 234
Testicle enlarged and pulpy 234
Scirrhus and Cancer of the Testicle 234
Testicle cartilaginous 235
Testicle bony 235
A Cyst adhering to a Testicle containing a Vena Medinensis 235
The Epidydimis ending in a Cul-de-sac 236
Stricture of the Vas Deferens 236

Testicles very small, and wasted 236
Diseased Appearances of the Spermatic Chord.
Spermatic Chord Scirrhous 237
Veins of the Spermatic Chord varicose 237
Water accumulated in the cellular Membrane of the Spermatic chord 237
A Sack containing water formed in the Spermatic chord 238
SYMPTOMS 238

CHAPTER XIX–DISEASED APPEARANCES IN THE FEMALE ORGANS 240

Inflammation of the Uterus 240
Malignant Ulcer of the Uterus 240
Scirrhous Enlargement of the Uterus 241
Tubercles of the Uterus 241
Polypus 242
The Inversion of the Uterus 243
Prolapsus Uteri 244
Stricture in the cavity of the Uterus 244
The Os Uteri contracted, and closed up 244
Uterus bony 244
The Uterus changed into an earthy Substance 245
A bony mass in the Cavity of the Uterus 245
Stones in the Cavity of the Uterus 245
Dead Foetus in the Uterus converted into an earthy Mass 245
Water in the Cavity of the Uterus 246
Hydatids in the Uterus 246
Rupture of the Uterus 247
Two Uteri 247
Natural Varieties in the Uterus 247
SYMPTOMS 248

CHAPTER XX–DISEASED APPEARANCES OF THE OVARIA 251

Inflammation of the Peritonaeal covering of the Ovaria 251

Inflammation of the substance of the Ovaria 251
Scirrhus of the Ovaria 251
Ovaria enlarged and changed into a pulpy Substance . . . 252
Ovaria Scrofulous 252
Dropsy of the Ovaria 252
The Ovaria changed into a fatty Substance with
Hair and Teeth 253
A Foetus in the Ovarium 255
Shrinking of the Ovaria 255
One Ovarium or both wanting 255
SYMPTOMS 256

CHAPTER XXI–DISEASED APPEARANCES OF
THE FALLOPIAN TUBES 257

Inflammation of the Fallopian Tubes 257
Adhesions 257
Dropsy of the Fallopian Tubes 257
The Fallopian tubes terminating in a Cul-de-sac 258
An Ovum in the Fallopian Tube 258
Hard Tumour growing from a Fallopian Tube 259
Diseased appearances of the round Ligaments 259
SYMPTOMS 259

CHAPTER XXII–DISEASED APPEARANCES OF
THE VAGINA 260

Inflammation of the Vagina 260
Adhesion of the Sides of the Vagina 260
Ulcers of the Vagina 260
Scirrhous Tumours in the Vagina 260
Inversion of the Vagina 261
The Vagina very short 262
The Vagina widened 262
The Vagina very narrow 262
SYMPTOMS 262

CHAPTER XXIII–DISEASED AND PRETERNATURAL
APPEARANCES OF THE EXTERNAL PARTS . . 264

The Hymen imperforated 264

The Clitoris enlarged 264
The Nymphae enlarged 265
The external Labia growing together 265

CHAPTER XXIV–DISEASED APPEARANCES OF THE BRAIN AND ITS MEMBRANES 266

Inflammation of the Dura Mater 266
Scrofulous Tumours connected with the Dura Mater . . . 267
Spongy Tumours growing from the Dura Mater 267
Bony Matter formed in the Dura Mater 267
Very strong Adhesions of the Dura Mater to the Cranium 268
Diseased appearances of the Tunica Arachnoides 268
Diseased Appearances of the Pia Mater.
Veins of the Pia Mater turgid with Blood 268
The Pia Mater inflamed 269
Scrofulous Tumours adhering to the Pia Mater 269
Air in the Vessels of the Pia Mater 269
Hydatids 270
A Part of the Pia Mater bony 270
Diseased Appearances in the Substance of the Brain.
Inflammation 270
Abscesses 271
Gangrene 271
The Brain very soft 271
The Brain very firm 272
A white firm Substance formed in the Brain 272
Encysted Tumours and Hydatids 272
Bony Tumours pressing upon the Brain 273
Bony Ridges irritating the Brain 273
Hydrocephalus 274
Water upon the Surface of the Brain, and between its Membranes 275
Blood effused or extravasated 276
Cavities in the Brain containing a serous Fluid 277
Aneurysm of the internal Carotid Arteries on the Side of the Sella Turcica 277
Diseased Appearances of the Plexus Choroides.
Little Bags in the Plexus Choroides 278

Round Tumours adhering to the Plexus Choroides 278
Diseased Appearances of the Pineal Gland.
Earthy Matter in the Pineal Gland 278
Pineal Gland said to be scirrhous 279
Water in the Pineal Gland 279
Diseased Appearances of the Pituitary Gland 279
Diseased Appearances of the Nerves 279
Mal-formations of the Brain 280
SYMPTOMS 280

PREFACE TO THE FIRST EDITION

SOME diseases consist only in morbib actions, but do not produce any change in the structure of parts; these do not admit of anatomical inquiry after death. There are other diseases, however, where alterations in the structure take place, and these become the proper subjects of anatomical examination.

The object of this work is to explain, more minutely than has hitherto been done, the changes of structure arising from morbid actions in some of the most important parts of the human body.

This, I hope, will be attended with some advantages to the general science of medicine, and ultimately to its practice. It is very much to be regretted that the knowledge of morbid structure does not lead with certainty to the knowledge of morbid actions, although the one is the effect of the other; yet surely it lays the most solid foundation for prosecuting such enquiries with success. In proportion, therefore, as we shall become acquainted with the changes produced in the structure of parts from diseased actions, we shall be more likely to make some progress towards a knowledge of the actions themselves, although it must be very slowly. The subject in itself is extremely difficult, because morbid actions are going on in the minute parts of an animal body excluded from observation; but still the examination of morbid structure is one of the most probable means of throwing light upon it.

A second advantage arising from the more attentive examination of morbid structure is, that we shall be able to distinguish between changes which may have some considerable resemblance to each other, and which have been generally confounded. This will ultimately lead to a more attentive observation of symptoms while morbid actions are taking place, and be the means of distinguishing disease with greater accuracy. When this has been done, it may, perhaps, produce a successful enquiry after the most proper method of treatment.

Another advantage arising from a more attentive observation of morbid structure is, that we shall be better fitted to detect diseased alterations in the organization of parts which are but little, or not at all known. This will lay the foundation of our inquiry into the diseases themselves, so that we shall add to our knowledge of the pathology of the body, and perhaps also to our knowledge of remedies.

A fourth advantage still from observing attentively morbid structure is, that theories taken up hastily about diseases will be occasionally corrected. The human mind is prone to form opinions upon every subject which is presented to it, but from a natural indolence is frequently averse to inquire into the circumstances which can alone form a sufficient ground for them. This is the most general cause of false opinions, which have not only pervaded medicine, but almost every other branch of knowledge. When, however, the mind shall be obliged to observe facts which cannot be reconciled with such opinions, it will be evident that the opinions are ill founded, and they will be laid aside. We grant, it does not always happen that men are induced to give up their opinions, or even to think them wrong, upon observing facts which do not agree with them, but surely it is the best means of producing this effect; and whatever change may be wrought on the individuals themselves, the world will be convinced, who have fewer prejudices to combat.

A person who previously had attended very accurately to symptoms, but was unacquainted with the disease, when he comes to examine the body after death, and finds some of the appearances that are described in this Treatise, will acquire a knowledge of the whole disease. He will be able to guide himself on such knowledge in similar cases, and also to inform others. It may, perhaps, too, lead him to a proper method of treatment.

When a person has become well acquainted with diseased appearances, he will be better able to make his remarks, in examining dead bodies, so as to judge more accurately how far the symptoms and the appearances agree with each other; he will be able also to give a more distinct account of what he has observed, so that his data will become a more accurate ground of reasoning for others.

The natural structure of the different parts of the human body has been very minutely examined, so that anatomy may be said to have arrived at a high pitch of perfection; but our knowledge of the changes of structure produced by disease, which may be called the Morbid Anatomy, is still very imperfect. Such changes have commonly been observed only in their more obvious appearances, and very seldom with much minuteness or accuracy of discrimination.

Any works explaining morbid structure which I have seen, are very different in their plan from the present: they either consist of cases containing an account of diseases and dissections collected together in periodical publications, without any natural connexion among each other; or consist of very large collections of cases, arranged according to some order. In some of these periodical works, the diseased structure has been frequently explained with a sufficient degree of accuracy, but in all the larger works it has been often described too generally. The descriptions too of the principal diseased appearances, have been sometimes obscured, by taking notice of smaller collateral circumstances, which had no connection with them or the diseases from whence they arose. Both of these faults too frequently occur, even in the stupendous work of Morgagni de Causis et Sedibus Morborum, upon which, when considered in all its parts, it would be difficult to bestow too high praise. Besides, the bulk of these very large collections prevents them from being generally in the possession of practitioners, and also renders them more difficult to consult.

In the present work we propose not to give cases; but simply an account of the morbid changes of structure which take place in the thoracic and abdominal viscera, in the organs of generation in both sexes, and in the brain. This will be done according to a local arrangement, very much in the same manner as if we were describing natural structure, and will be accompanied with observations upon morbid actions which may occasionally arise. My situation has given me more than the ordinary opportunities of examining morbid structure. Dr. Hunter's collection contains a very large number of preparations exhibiting morbid appearances, which I can have recourse to at any time for examination. Being physician to a large hospital, and engaged in teaching anatomy, I have also very frequent opportunities of examining diseases in dead bodies. This work will therefore chiefly contain an account of the morbid appearances which I have seen myself; but I shall also take advantage of what has been observed by others. It is intended to comprehend an account of the most common, as well as many of the very rare appearances of disease in the vital and more important parts of the human body. From the nature of this undertaking it is evident, that it must be progressive: some appearances of disease will be observed in future, with which we are at present totally unacquainted, and others which we know very little of now, will afterwards be known perfectly.

Although I have ventured to lay this work before the Public, yet I am very sensible of its imperfections. Some appearances are described which I have only had an opportunity of seeing once, and which, therefore, may be supposed to be described less fully and exactly than if I had been able to make repeated examinations. There are others which I have seen long before I had formed any idea of this undertaking, and which I may be supposed to have observed less accurately than if I had had a particular object in view. There are others still, which I only have had an opportunity of examining in preparations. In some of these, certain appearances may be supposed to be lost, which might have been observed had they been examined recently after death. All of these are sources of inaccuracy, which may be said in some degree to be unavoidable. I have endeavoured, however, to be accurate; and if the Public should approve of my plan, I shall be very careful, by the addition of new materials, and by repeated observations, to render this publication more perfect.

PREFACE TO THE SECOND EDITION

A SECOND EDITION of this Treatise is now offered to the Public. It is considerably enlarged, and I hope more correct than the former. The additions are principally derived from what I have remarked myself; but they are also taken from the observations of others, and more especially from those of Dr. Soemmerring, Professor of Medicine in the University of Mayence, one of the most distinguished anatomists in Germany. He was pleased to think so favourably of my attempt to improve the knowledge of diseased appearances in the human body, as to translate the first Edition of the Morbid Anatomy into the German language, and to add to it many new Cases, and copious Notes. It has given me the most sincere satisfaction, to find that our observations and opinions coincide so much with those of each other. Had the plan of my work been different, I might have derived much more assistance from the valuable labours of Professor Soemmerring, but many of the additions which he has made do not strictly fall within it.

To the Morbid Appearances I have attempted to subjoin the Symptoms connected with them. This part of the undertaking is attended with many difficulties, and I feel, very sensibly, how much the execution of it stands in need of the kind indulgence of the public. If this work shall ever come to another Edition, I hope to be able to render the account of symptoms less imperfect.

The difficulties which attend an attempt to ascertain the symptoms of diseases, are derived from various sources. The same symptoms are not uniformly connected with the same changes of morbid structure in the body. In many cases too the symptoms are nearly the same, where the morbid changes of structure are very different. This is particularly exemplified in diseases of the brain, and of the heart. Patients often explain very imperfectly their feelings, partly from the natural deficiency of language, and partly from being misled by preconceived opinions about the nature of their complaints. Medical men also, in examining into the symptoms of diseases, sometimes put their questions inaccurately, and not unfrequently mislead patients into a false description, from some opinion about the disease which they have too hastily adopted. All of these are formidable difficulties, which obstruct the progress of our knowledge of the symptoms of disease; but the accumulated observations of many individuals will probably, at length, in a great measure overcome them.

In describing the symptoms of disease, I have not entered into a minute detail. This belongs properly to the plan of a writer, who proposes to take a full view of any particular disease. I have mentioned those symptoms only which are most constant, and most strongly characteristic of the diseases to which they belong. Many diseased appearances are described in this work, to which there are added no corresponding symptoms; and this depends upon different causes. The first is, that there are many morbid changes of structure in the body, the corresponding symptoms of which are not ascertained. The second is, that many morbid changes of structure are produced by causes which disturb the constitution so little, as to be attended with symptoms too slightly marked for observation. The third and last is, that the symptoms belonging to some diseased appearances, fall so immediately under the cognizance of the eye, or of the touch, as to be included in a description of the diseased appearances themselves, and to render any further account of them superfluous.

The account of symptoms is placed at the end of each chapter, after the description of the diseased appearances, that the anatomical part of the work may not be interrupted. In a very few instances, however, the account of the symptoms has not been separated from the anatomical description of the morbid appearances, viz. where so little of the symptoms was known as not to admit of a distinct account being given of them.

Besides an account of morbid appearances, a few cases of malformation are blended in this work. They do not strictly fall within its plan; I have, therefore, added only a few, which are important, and which have almost all occurred to my own observation.

London
Nov. 20, 1797.

ADVERTISEMENT TO THE THIRD EDITION

FOR the last seven years I have been so much engaged in the practical duties of my Profession, as only to have had occasional opportunities of inspecting dead bodies. I have therefore, scarcely been able to make any additions to this Work, but I have made such corrections of it, as more reflection and experience have suggested to me, and I hope it will be found to be considerably improved.

The Second Edition of this treatise was translated about three years ago, by Dr. Ferrall, into the French language. The translation is made with great fidelity; but, as it is neither accompanied with Notes, nor with the addition of any new cases, I have not been able to derive any advantage from it, in preparing this Third Edition for the Press.

LONDON
Feb. 1, 1807.

CHAPTER I

DISEASED APPEARANCES OF THE PERICARDIUM

Inflammation of the Pericardium

THE pericardium, or the membrane which surrounds the heart like a bag, and is reflected upon its surface, giving it a smooth external covering, is liable to inflammation. This is not a very common disease, although it happens sufficiently often to afford frequent opportunities of examining its effects after death. The disease, from its nature, cannot be confined to any particular periods of life; yet from what I have seen, I should believe that it takes place more commonly when the body has been for some time in its adult state, than either in childhood or advanced age.

In inflammation of the pericardium, the membrane is frequently thicker than in its natural state, and is also a little more pulpy. This change depends upon additional matter being thrown into the membrane by the increased action of the small vessels which are distributed upon it. It is also crowded with a very unusual number of minute vessels, which contain florid blood. Upon the inside of the pericardium there is a layer of a yellowish pulpy matter, which commonly does not adhere firmly to it, but may be easily separated. It generally extends over the whole of its inner surface, and varies a good deal in its thickness. In some instances it is as thin as a wafer, and in others as thick as a half-crown. In this matter, which is lining the pericardium, there is frequently to be seen a slight red appearance, from small blood vessels which are ramifying through it; but these are most distinctly detected by filling them with the fine injection. They are sometimes numerous, and may be clearly traced passing from the pericardium into the pulpy matter; in which I have also seen small spots of florid blood. These newly formed vessels afford a very convincing proof of this extravasated matter possessing a living principle, for one cannot imagine that blood vessels would shoot into, and form a number of new branches in a substance which is dead (1). Upon its inner surface, this matter very frequently throws out little irregular processes, giving the appearance of lace-work, and junctions are often formed between that portion of it lining the pericardium, which is reflected like a bag, and that other portion lying upon the pericardium, which is the immediate covering of the heart. This matter has a very close resemblance, both in colour and structure, to the coagulable lymph of the blood, and is probably nothing else than this substance separated from the blood by a particular action of the small vessels of the pericardium.

At the same time that this layer of pulpy matter is thrown out upon the inner surface of the pericardium, there is accumulated in its cavity more or less of a brownish or yellowish fluid. There is sometimes only a few ounces of it; at other times more than a pint. In it are floating, loose shreds of the pulpy matter formerly described, and there is also occasionally some mixture of pus. This fluid resembles in its properties the serum of the blood, and has commonly been considered as the serum.

Inflammation of the pericardium sometimes advances to form pus, although rarely. Of this I have seen one instance. The pericardium was much thickened, was inflamed, and lined with coagulable lymph; but there was no sign of ulceration in any part of it. This last circumstance will be more particularly taken notice of, when we come to speak of the diseased appearances of the pleura. The pericardium in this case, contained more than a quart of common pus. When that part of the pericardium is inflamed which forms the immediate covering of the heart, the muscular substance of the latter is occasionally inflamed to some depth.

When the pericardium, or any other membrane lining a circumscribed cavity, is inflamed, and a layer of coagulable lymph is formed upon its surface, there is a peculiar disposition given to the coagulable lymph by the action of the small vessels which pour it out. This peculiar disposition is its tendency to immediate coagulation. As soon as the coagulable lymph is thrown out upon

1. This is an argument used by Mr. Hunter, in support of the living principle of blood.

an inflamed surface, one must suppose that it immediately coagulates. If it did not immediately coagulate, but remained for some time fluid, as in the spontaneous separation of the constituent parts of the blood in a bason after common bleeding, then the coagulable lymph would form a small cake at the bottom of the serum, easily moveable from one part of the cavity to another, and would not form a layer adhering to the surface of the inflamed membrane.

The serum is generally in a much larger quantity than could take place in consequence of its mere spontaneous separation from the coagulable lymph which is spread upon the surface of the inflamed membrane. The blood vessels, therefore, which are distributed in the layer of the coagulable lymph, would seem to pour out some quantity of serum. While the inflammation is receding, and the coagulable lymph is changing into adhesions, the serum is generally taken up from the cavity; and this effect must be supposed to be produced by the action of absorbent vessels. The membrane of adhesions must therefore have absorbent vessels belonging to it, which have probably been formed by the elongation or growth of the absorbents of the inflamed membrane, shooting into the coagulable lymph.

Besides serum, we have mentioned that pus is sometimes found in an inflamed circumscribed cavity. When this is the case, it seems extremely probable that the small arteries, distributed in the layer of the coagulable lymph, have poured out the pus. This, I believe, has not hitherto been thought of; but it is difficult to conceive under these circumstances any other source from whence the pus is derived. If the pus be supposed to be formed by the arteries which ramify in the inflamed membrane itself, then it must transude through a layer of coagulable lymph, which often is of considerable thickness, before it accumulates in the cavity. This, however, is not likely; and as arteries pass from the original membrane into the layer of the coagulable lymph, it becomes more reasonable to suppose that pus is formed by the arteries distributed in the coagulable lymph, than in the original membrane itself.

Adhesions of the Pericardium to the Heart

In opening dead bodies, adhesions of the pericardium to the

heart, are not uncommonly found. The adhesion is sometimes at different spots; at other times is extended over the whole surface. It either consists of a thin membrane, or of a more solid matter. When it is a thin membrane, it resembles exactly the common cellular membrane of the body; and when the matter is solid, it differs only a little from the coagulable lymph of the blood, recently thrown out upon an inflamed surface. Whether the adhesion be in the one way or the other, the matter of the adhesion is in both cases capable of being rendered vascular by injection. The adhesion too is in both cases formed from the pulpy matter formerly explained, for I have oftener than once had an opportunity of tracing its gradual changes into each. Such adhesions are to be considered as the consequence of inflammation, and shew that an inflammation of the pericardium may be survived. They connect the pericardium in different cases, more closely or loosely to the surface of the heart; and where the connection is close, the inflammation has probably been more recent; where it is loose, the inflammation has probably been of older date, so that time has been given for the adhesions to be elongated by the motion of the heart.

Dropsy of the Pericardium

This disease is not uncommon, and I believe is most frequent at an advanced period of life. I have seen it, however, in persons considerably under the age of thirty: and it probably also happens occasionally in childhood, I have seen oftener than once both anasarca and ascites in children under twelve years old, which is as improbable as the accumulation of water in the pericardium. Water is sometimes found accumulated in the pericardium, while there is none in any other cavity; but generally it is accompanied with the accumulation of water in the other cavities of the thorax.

This water varies a good deal in quantity, amounting in some cases hardly to two ounces, and in others to more than a pint. Although the quantity be large which may happen to be accumulated, yet the pericardium is never very much stretched; but it always appears as if it could contain a greater quantity. It is probable, therefore, that the pericardium may really grow so as to keep pace with the accumulation; and this would seem to be necessary, in order that the heart may have room for dilating its several cavities.

The fluid, which is accumulated, is of a brown colour, having a darker or lighter shade in different cases, and resembles in its properties the serum of the blood. If the person should happen at the same time to have jaundice, then the fluid has a yellow tinge from the bile. It has, however, frequently a yellowish colour, like the serum, without here being any reason to suppose that bile has been circulating with the blood.

Scrofulous Tumours in the Pericardium

I had once an opportunity of seeing two or three scrofulous tumours, growing within the cavity of the pericardium, one of which was nearly as large as a walnut. They consisted of a white, soft matter, somewhat resembling curd or new cheese. The pericardium is a very unusual part of the body to be attacked by scrofula, and therefore this must be considered as a very rare appearance of disease.

The Pericardium almost dry

I have twice found (and it has been seen much oftener by an anatomist (2), whose authority is of great weight) the pericardium so changed as to resemble a common ox's bladder in some degree dried; or like a common pericardium which had been for some time exposed to the air. As the thorax and abdomen were entire in both cases, no opening whatever having been made into either, this effect could not arise from evaporation. Were this capable of taking place, the appearance here noticed, would be very unusual in examining dead bodies, and the internal parts generally would be effected by the influence of the same cause. It must be considered therefore as the effect of a process which was going on during life. The cause of this appearance is either a defect in the action of the exhalant vessels of the pericardium, so that the fluid

2. Mr. Hunter.

which naturally lubricates this part, is not secreted in the proper quantity: or it is an increased action of the absorbent vessels of the pericardium, by which the lubricating fluid is taken up in larger proportion than it is deposited by the exhalant arteries.

The Pericardium cartilaginous, and bony

A portion of the pericardium has in some instances been observed to be converted into cartilage (3), and in others into bone (4), but both of these changes are very uncommon.

I had an opportunity lately of examining an instance of the latter sort, in which the ossific process had spread over a considerable portion of the pericardium. A cartilaginous state of the pericardium has not fallen under my own observation.

The Pericardium wanting

A few instances have occurred, in which the pericardium has been wanting, from a defect in the original formation. When this deficiency takes place, the heart appears perfectly bare and distinct to the eye, upon removing the sternum and the cartilaginous extremities of the ribs. The external surface of the different cavities and blood vessels of the heart is seen as distinctly as when the pericardium is laid open in the natural structure of these parts. A close and uniform adhesion of the pericardium to the heart has sometimes been mistaken for this malformation, but they are very different from each other. When there is a close adhesion of the pericardium to the heart, the external surface of the different cavities and blood vessels of this organ does not come into view, upon removing the sternum and a part of the ribs. The whole of this appearance is as completely hid as in the healthy structure. It is only when the adhesion is removed by dissection that the external surface of the heart and its blood vessels comes into view. When there is an adhesion of the pericardium to the heart, this membrane adheres at the same time closely to the tendinous part of the diaphragm; but when there is an original want of the

---

3. See Morgagni de Causis et Sedibus Morborum, Epist. XXII, Aft. 10.
4. See Bonetus, Tom. I. p. 583.

pericardium, the heart lies loose in the cavity of the chest, having no connection whatever with the diaphragm, and is covered by the pleura, like the lungs. I have had an opportunity of seeing once an example of a want of the pericardium, and have described it in the Medical and Chirurgical transactions (5).

SYMPTOMS

The symptoms attending inflammation of the pericardium, cannot be distinguished in practice from inflammation of the substance of the heart. Whenever the inflammation of the pericardium is violent, the muscular substance of the heart is inflamed to some depth, and therefore the inflammation of both parts are often blended together. The symptoms, which have been observed, are the general affection of the system known by the name of Symptomatic Fever; pain in the region of the heart, which is often, but not always attended with palpitations, and with an irregular pulse; cough; difficulty of breathing; and sometimes syncope.

The symptoms attending adhesions of the pericardium to the heart, are not so clearly marked as to be well distinguished in practice. When the adhesions are partial and long, so that the heart can enjoy a free play within the pericardium, probably little or no inconvenience is felt. But when the adhesions are close, and extend generally over the surface of the heart, the following symptoms have been observed, viz. a sense of oppression, and sometimes of pain in the situation of the heart; a pulse often irregular and intermittent; difficulty of breathing, and sometimes a dry cough.

When water is accumulated in the pericardium, the symptoms are found to resemble very much those belonging to hydrothorax, and have not been clearly distinguished from them by authors. These symptoms will be afterwards mentioned when we come to hydrothorax. It may perhaps serve as some imperfect ground of distinction between the two diseases, that the feeling of oppression is more accurately confined to the situation of the heart, and

5. See page 91, Vol. I.

the heart is more disturbed in its functions, in dropsy of the pericardium, than in hydrothorax. It ought at the same time to be remarked, that the two diseases are often blended, in which case, these grounds of distinction cannot be applied.

The case of scrofulous tumours growing upon the inside of the pericardium, which I have described, was combined with tubercles of the lungs; and the person died with the common symptoms of pulmonary consumption. Nothing occurred which led to any suspicion of a disease in the pericardium. It seems to me reasonable to suppose, that when scrofulous tumours grow in the pericardium, there will hardly be any inconvenience felt while they are small; but when they enlarge very much in size, they will necessarily prevent the full dilation of the heart, and disturb its functions. This, however, will probably be very difficult to be distinguished from the disturbance produced by other causes, which must in the same manner impede the free action of the heart; as, for instance, the accumulation of water in the pericardium.

The symptoms produced by a defect of the lubricating fluid in the pericardium, are at present unknown.

CHAPTER II

DISEASED APPEARANCES OF THE HEART

Inflammation of the Heart

INFLAMMATION of the substance of the heart is a rare disease, and is most commonly connected with an inflammation of the pericardium. When the pericardium covering its surface is inflamed, the inflammation sometimes passes a little way into the substance of the heart. That part of it becomes much more crowded with small vessels than in its natural state, and there are sometimes to be seen in it a few spots of extravasated blood. The substance of the heart may, however, be inflamed, without inflammation of the pericardium. I recollect an instance of this sort, where no marks of inflammation could be observed in that membrane, but where there was a little more water than usual in its cavity.

Authors have mentioned cases of abscesses and ulcers (6) of the heart, but these I am persuaded are extremely rare. It happens still more rarely that the heart becomes mortified, although this diseased state of it has also been observed (7).

White Spot upon the Surface of the Heart

In opening dead bodies there is very often to be seen upon the surface of the heart, a white opaque spot like a thickening of the pericardium. This is sometimes not broader than a six-pence; at other times as broad as a crown-piece. It is most commonly on the surface of the right ventricle, and is rarely to be seen either on the surface of the left ventricle, or of the auricles, although it is

6. Vide Morgagni, Epist. XXV. Artic. 17. Vide Bonet. Tom. I. p. 849; and also Lieutaud, Tom. II. p. 27.
7. Vide Lieutaud, Tom. II. p. 33.

occasionally on both.

It consists of an adventitious membrane, formed on a portion of the pericardium which covers the heart, and may easily be dissected off, so as to leave the pericardium entire. It is an appearance, I believe, of no consequence whatever, and is so very common, that it can hardly be considered as a disease.

Polypus

This has been considered by the older anatomists, as a very common and a very fatal disease. By many of the moderns it has been rejected as a disease altogether. It consists of a mass of the coagulable lymph, which fills up some of the large cavities of the heart, particularly the ventricles, and extends into the neighbouring large vessels.

The coagulable lymph is of a yellowish white colour, sometimes of a very yellow colour, and has considerable firmness. It fills up the cavity completely, or nearly so, in which it is found; and in the ventricles it shoots out processes among the fasciculi of the muscular fibres. From this circumstance probably, it has derived its name. It also extends into the larger arteries which arise from the ventricles, and is often moulded to the semi-lunar valves at their origin. The examples of this appearance which it has occurred to me to observe, have been chiefly in preparations, and had undoubtedly taken place after death. In order that the cavities of the heart be free for the transmission of blood; and if any one of its cavities should be plugged up, the circulation would necessarily be stopped altogether. A polypus, however, plugs up the cavity of the heart in which it is formed so entirely, as to prevent the circulation. It may be said, perhaps, that polypi are formed gradually, and that the circulation is carried on for some time, although very imperfectly. We have no evidence, however, of coagula of blood being formed in the ordinary circulation, where there is a healthy structure of the parts concerned in this function. When polypi are examined, there is the same sort of appearance throughout their whole substance; which shews that the whole coagulum had been formed at the same time. Both of those circumstances seem to contradict very strongly the opinion, that polypi are formed during life. When polypi are formed, I believe that the coagulation of the blood does not take place very quickly after death. They are without any admixture of the red globules of blood, and therefore the blood has been sufficiently long in coagulating to allow the globules to separate from the other parts, in consequence of their greater specific gravity.

The ordinary coagulations of the blood, which commonly do not fill up very fully the cavities of the heart (although instances occasionally occur of this sort) take place pretty soon after death, because the red particles of the blood are generally arrested in the coagulum. It may be worth while to remark, that there is sometimes found a portion of a coagulum in one of the ventricles of a yellow colour, and with an oily appearance, so as to resemble exactly fat. There is, however, no admixture of oil in it, and it possesses all the ordinary properties of the coagulable lymph. The yellow colour of a coagulum sometimes depends on a portion of the bile having circulated with the blood during life, as in cases of jaundice; but it takes place also when there is no reason to suppose that bile is mixed with the blood.

Aneurysm of the Heart

It sometimes happens, although I believe very rarely, that the heart becomes aneurysmal. This disease consists in a part of it being dilated into a pouch, which is commonly more or less filled with coagulated blood. Of this disease I have only seen one instance. The apex of the left ventricle was dilated into a pouch large enough to contain a small orange, was much thinner than in the healthy structure, and was lined with a thick, white, opaque, membrane. There was hardly contained in it any coagulated blood; but the quantity of the coagulated blood, in an aneurysm, depends commonly on the size of the bag.

This disease most probably arose from the muscular structure at the apex of the ventricle becoming weaker than in any other part, so that when the ventricle contracted upon the blood, it was pushed against the weakened part, which was not fully able to resist its impetus, and therefore was gradually dilated – had the strength of the apex of the left ventricle been in due proportion to that of the other parts, it would seem impossible that the aneurysmal swelling should ever have taken place.

Aneurysm of the Arch of the Aorta

The most frequent situation of aneurysm within the cavity of the thorax, is at the arch of the aorta. In this disease the arch of the aorta is much enlarged beyond its usual size, sometimes forming an uniform tumour; at other times there are smaller aneurysmal swellings rising out of the larger one. This enlargement of the artery, if very considerable, is more or less filled with coagulated blood, which is disposed in concentric laminae. The coats of the dilated artery are nearly of the same thickness with those in its natural state; and therefore in proportion as the swelling increases, new matter must be deposited in the coats of the artery. This new matter would seem to be deposited with a view to prevent the artery from being so soon ruptured as it would be otherwise, and is formed by the action of the vasa vasorum. A portion of the new matter may perhaps also be formed by the action of the parts immediately in contact with the artery.

The coats of the artery, both at the place where the aneurysm is formed, and near it, are considerably altered from their natural structure. They are more readily divisable into different layers, than where the artery is sound, and have often formed in them spots of bony matter. These spots are frequently of a yellowish colour, and are formed either in the internal membrane of the artery, or immediately behind it.

The coats of the artery in the neighborhood of the aneurysm, are often found to be very irregular in their texture, being in some places transparent and thin, in others thick and opaque; and there is sometimes the appearance of a double internal membrane. The same sort of structure is also to be found in the coats of the aneurysm itself. The arteries near an aneurysm are diseased to a greater or less extent in different persons; but I do not recollect one instance in which they were totally free from disease.

The disease sometimes ends fatally, by the enlarged artery bursting, and the blood, escaping into the cavity of the pericardium; but it very often has a further progress; the swelling of the aneurysm gradually increases, till at length it presses against the sternum, and the cartilaginous extremities of some of the ribs. This pressure occasions a portion of the sternum and the ribs to be absorbed, and the tumor is thereby perceived externally. The absorption of the sternum and ribs goes on very gradually, and is not accompanied with the formation of pus. The tumour gradually increases in size, till perhaps it is as large as a child's head at birth; a part of the skin becomes in some measure dead, and cracks from distention at the highest point of the tumor; a portion of the coagulated blood is forced out by the impetus of the circulation, and the person is cut off instantaneously. The blood sometimes oozes out slowly, and the person sinks gradually under its loss.

Aneurysms at the arch of the aorta, as well as in every other part of the arterial system, arise from the coats of the artery being previously diseased, which are thereby unable to resist sufficiently the impetus of blood that strikes against them. This is obvious, both from the diseased structure of the coats of an aneurysm itself, and of the artery in its neighbourhood.

I have also found very frequently, diseased appearances in the arch of the aorta, which had not advanced far enough to produce aneurysms. These consist in little white opaque spots being formed in the inner membrane of the artery, and in its coats being more easily separable from each other than in the healthy state.

The reason why aneurysms take place more frequently in the arch of the aorta, than in any other part of the arterial system, is its curvature, which exposes it to the full impetus of the blood propelled by the strength of the left ventricle. Aneurysms hardly ever happen in the pulmonary artery, because there is no arch formed by the pulmonary artery, and the blood readily passes by two large branches into the substance of the lungs.

Aneurysms in the arch of the aorta, as well as in every other part of the arterial system, happen much more rarely in women than in men. This arises from two causes. The one is, that women, from their sedentary life, are less liable to an increased impetus of blood, occasioned by excited circulation; the other is, that the arteries in this sex appear to be less liable to these diseased alterations of structure, which predispose to aneurysm.

Ossification of the Coronary Arteries of the Heart

The coronary arteries are occasionally ossified in a greater or less degree. This state of them is, I believe, generally accompanied with ossified portions of the aorta at its origin, and sometimes with ossification of the semi-lunar valves.

Ossification of the Semi-lunar Valves

The three semi-lunar valves at the origin of the aorta, or of the pulmonary artery, are often found diseased. The disease very commonly consists in the deposition of a bony or earthy matter, and would seem to be formed by a morbid action of some very minute vessels which are distributed through the substance of the valves. These vessels are so small, as not to contain, in their natural state, the red globules of the blood.

Semi-lunar Valves thick and opaque

It frequently happens that the semi-lunar valves are considerably thickened, and of an opaque white colour: in this case, the coats of the artery in the neighbourhood, I believe, are commonly thickened and diseased.

Rupture of the Valves

There is a preparation in Dr. Hunter's collection, where one of the semi-lunar valves is thickened, having at the same time little tenacity, and in which a considerable rupture had taken place. It is very rare that such an occurrence happens, and in the present instance the rupture was so large, that I believe it must have proved almost immediately fatal.

Valves between the Auricles and the Ventricles ossified

The valvular apparatus between the auricles and ventricles, is liable to the formation of bony and earthy matter in it, as are also the valves which are situated at the origin of the two large arteries, but by no means so frequently. What this depends upon, it is very difficult to determine. These valves may perhaps be considered as belonging more to the venal than the arterial system, and it is certain that ossification takes place very seldom in veins, although very often in arteries.

The same Valves thick and opaque

The valvular apparatus between the auricles and ventricles is also occasionally thickened, having lost all its transparency, and having an opaque white colour. The chordae tendineae likewise become thicker than natural; and the internal membrane lining the ventricles is frequently at the same time a good deal thickened, appearing like a firm white membrane. Under such circumstances the heart is often found to be considerably enlarged beyond its usual size.

I have also seen the valvular apparatus between the auricle and the ventricle, in a state of inflammation, and covered with a layer of coagulable lymph: but this I believe to be very uncommon.

Rupture of the Heart

It sometimes happens, and I believe chiefly in those who are advanced in life, that the heart at some part becomes thinner, and upon any great exertion bursts. The blood escapes into the cavity of the pericardium, and the person is instantly destroyed.

Of this accident I have one instance only; but have heard from the best authority of another. They both happened to men; and I mention this circumstance, because men appear to be more subject to diseases of the heart and blood vessels than women. It is probable that persons dying from this cause have, on account of the suddenness of their death, been supposed to die of apoplexy.

Blood in the Pericardium, without a Rupture of the Heart

Cases have occurred, although very rarely, in which a large quantity of blood has been accumulated in the cavity of the pericardium, but where no rupture could be discovered after the most diligent search, either in the heart itself, or in any of its vessels. This appears very wonderful, and not at all what any person would expect *a priori.* Upon the supposition of there being no rupture, two conjectures only have occurred to me about the manner in which such an effect has taken place, and they are both attended with considerable difficulty.

The one is, that the vessels upon the surface of the heart, may have lost a part of the compactness of their texture, so that the blood may have escaped through their coats by transudation. The other is, that blood may have been thrown out by the extremities of the small vessels opening upon the surface, of that portion chiefly of the pericardium which forms the immediate covering of the heart, from their orifices having been to a very uncommon degree relaxed (8).

Malformation of the Heart

It also happens, although I believe very rarely, that the heart is so imperfectly formed as to allow of life being continued for some length of time, in a very uncomfortable state, but to be ultimately the cause of death. There are two cases of this sort described by the late Dr. Hunter (9), and there is one specimen of this malformation preserved in his collection. The malformation preserved in the collection, consists in the right ventricle of the heart being extremely small, and the pulmonary artery being very small also which arises from it. At its origin from the right ventricle it is completely impervious. The ductus arteriosus is open, but forms likewise a small canal, and terminates in the left branch of the pulmonary artery. The right auricle is larger than it naturally is, from the frequent accumulation of blood in it; and the communication between the two auricles, by means of the foramen ovale, is much larger than usual. The child, in whom this malformation was found, had its skin of a very dark colour, and had very laborious respiration, with violent action of the heart. It lived only thirteen days.

In another case related by Dr. Hunter, the pulmonary artery

8. See Med. Observations, Vol. 4. p. 330. Memoirs of Med. Society, Vol. 1. p. 238.
9. Vid, Medical Observations, Vol. 6. p. 291.

was very small, especially at its origin, and there was a deficiency in the septum cordis, at the basis of the heart, large enough to allow a small thumb to pass through it. The person in whom this malformation of the heart was found, lived about thirteen years. He never had a fresh complexion, but it was always dark, or tending to black. He was often seized with fits, especially when there was any hurry upon his spirits, or there had been any brisk motion of his body.

It is obvious that in these deviations from the natural structure, too small a quantity of blood must pass through the lungs to receive the benefit of respiration, and that this will be more or less according to the degree of the deviation. The blood will from this cause be of a dark colour, as it is well known that it receives the florid hue from the influence of the air upon it in the lungs. Hence the colour of the skin must be necessarily dark, and this will be increased when the blood is accumulated more than usual in the veins. It is natural to think that in such structures of the heart, the circulation will be carried on with much more difficulty when it is excited beyond its usual standard. This may even be supposed to be encreased to such a degree as to produce fits, which happened in one of the Cases.

There is an example also in Dr. Hunter's collection of a heart from a child, which had a hole in the septum ventriculorum at the basis of the heart, large enough to allow a goose quill readily to pass through it. The child was still born at six months, and the hole in the septum evidently arose from original malformation. This too is described by Dr. Hunter, in the sixth volume of the Medical Observations. An instance somewhat similar to this has been published by Dr. Pulteney, in the third volume of the Medical Transactions; the person to whom this monstrosity belonged, lived to near fourteen years of age.

A very singular malformation of the heart, in a child about two months old, came some time ago into my possession, which I shall describe in this place. The aorta in this heart arose out of the right ventricle, and the pulmonary artery out of the left. There was no communication between the one vessel and the other, except through the small remains of the ductus arteriosus, which was just large enough to admit a crow quill. The foramen ovale was little more closed than in a child newly born. The heart was of the common size for a child of two months old, and, except for the circumstances which have been stated, had nothing remarkable in its structure. In this child a florid blood must have been always circulating between the lungs and the left side of the heart, except for the admixture of the dark blood which passed through the small communication of the foramen ovale; and a dark blood must have been always circulating between the right side of the heart and the general mass of the body, except for the very small quantity of florid blood which passed into the aorta by the remains of the ductus arteriosus. Life must, therefore, have been supported for a very considerable length of time with hardly any florid blood distributed over the body. I regret extremely that I have only been able to collect a very imperfect account of the child when alive. The child had a most unusually livid skin, which arose from the very small proportion of the florid blood in the general circulation. The surface of the child's body felt colder than that of a child properly formed and in good health; the respiration was natural. When any similar malformation shall occur, it could be wished that the heat of the surface of the body, and of the internal parts, were measured accurately by a thermometer. The heat of the internal parts will be most conveniently measured by putting a small thermometer into the rectum (10).

Heart Enlarged

The heart is sometimes found very much enlarged in its size, but without any apparent disease in its structure. The muscular parietes are generally as thin and sometimes even thinner than in a heart of the common size. Its cavities are filled with blood, partly fluid, and partly concreted into a loose coagulum.

Hydatids adhering to the Heart

Hydatids (11) have occasionally been found adhering to the

10. This very singular malformation of the heart was given to me by Dr. Wollaston, of St. Edmundsbury, who took much trouble in endeavouring to collect information about the child, but without the desired success.

11. See Morgagni, Epist. XXV. Art. 15.

heart; but I have not met myself with any instances of this sort. They do not appear to be of the same kind in every part of the body; but their nature will be explained particularly, when I come to describe the diseased appearances of the liver and kidneys.

A Portion of the Heart bony, or earthy

A portion of the heart has been observed to be converted into bone (12). Earthy matter has also been found deposited in the muscular substance of the heart (13). Neither of these appearances has come under my own observation, and they are to be looked upon as very uncommon.

SYMPTOMS

The symptoms which attend inflammation of the heart are very much the same with those which belong to inflammation of the pericardium, viz, symptomatic fever; pain in the situation of the heart; palpitations; an irregular pulse; cough; difficulty of breathing; and often syncope. It would seem probable that the last symptom is principally connected with inflammation of the substance of the heart, and perhaps it may not be found in a pure inflammation of the pericardium. The two diseases, however, are very commonly blended together.

The symptoms which attend aneurysm of the heart, are similar to those which belong to aneurysm of the arch of the aorta.

The chief symptom which attends aneurysm of the arch of the aorta, in an early stage of the disease, is a strong pulsation in the chest. The pulsation is commonly at the same time visible to the eye, when the chest is exposed to view. We are not to conclude, however, from this symptom, only, that there is certainly an aneurysm. I have felt the same kind of pulsation in other cases; as for instance, where the pericardium was found strongly to adhere to the heart; where was a slight inflammation upon the surface of the heart, with a little more water than usual in the pericardium;

12. See Morgagni, Epist. XXVII. Art. 16. See also Medical Communications, Vol. 1. p. 228.

13. See Bonetus, Tom. I. p. 820, and p. 875.

and where a morbid enlargement had taken place in the heart without any aneurysmal swelling. But when an aneurysm of the arch of the aorta has advanced to a large size, a tumour begins to be formed externally, accompanied with a strong pulsation. This I believe belongs only to aneurysm, and becomes the most decided characteristic of this disease. The pulse at the wrist in aneurysm of the arch of the aorta is sometimes irregular; but often no irregularity can be felt in it. There is generally more or less a pain in the aneurysmal tumour, or in some other part of the chest. Difficulty of breathing upon taking exercise also commonly attends this disease, which is increased in proportion as the disease advances.

Ossification of the coronary arteries would seem to produce, or to be intimately connected with the symptoms which constitute angina pectoris. These consist of a pain which shoots from the middle of the sternum across the left breast, and passes down the left arm, to near the elbow, somtimes even to the wrist of the left hand. In a few cases the pain has been known to shoot across the right breast as well as the left, and to pass down the right arm, either to near the elbow or the wrist. It is excited by walking, more especially up an ascent, and by any considerable emotion of the mind (14).

The symptoms, which are produced by a diseased alteration in the structure of the valves of the heart, are not so distinct as to be clearly discriminated in practice. They consist of difficulty of breathing; of occasional palpitations; of a weak and often an irregular pulse; and in some cases there has been observed a disposition of fainting. No observations have yet been made by which practitioners may be led to conjecture what set of valves is diseased.

The symptoms which have been noticed as attending a gradual effusion of blood into the pericardium, are a great degree of faintness; difficulty of breathing; much anxiety and oppression; a dull pain, and a sense of weight behind the sternum. To these a cold clammy sweat has been observed to succeed, and to spread over the body.

---

14. See an excellent treatise upon this subject by Dr. Parry.

When the heart is much enlarged, the disease is attended with palpitations. These may not only be felt by the hand, when applied to the left side, but may often be perceived by the eye, even when the chest is covered with the ordinary clothing. In one or two instances, I have known the pulse at the wrist to beat with an unusual degree of vigour, but much more commonly the pulse is feeble and irregular. The muscular parietes of the heart being generally thin in proportion to the enlarged size of its cavities, the heart has little power to propel an increased quantity of blood into the more distant branches of the arterial system. At times there is much difficulty of breathing; and there is a purplish hue of the cheeks and lips. This colour is more deep in its tinge at one time than another, according as the blood has been transmitted with more or less difficulty through the lungs. The causes which produce a morbid growth of the heart are but little known; one of them would seem to be rheumatism attacking this organ (15).

The symptoms produced by the formation of hydatids, in the cavity of the pericardium are not distinctly known; but they cannot be supposed to differ much from those of water in the pericardium. In a case related by Morgagni, the patient was subject to fainting.

When a part of the heart is converted into an earthy matter or bone, no morbid symptoms whatever have, in some cases, been observed; and in others there has been palpitation of the heart, with difficulty of breathing.

---

15. Dr. Pitcairn has observed this in several cases.

CHAPTER III

DISEASED APPEARANCES IN THE CAVITY OF THE THORAX

Inflammation

THE pleura, or the membrane which lines the cavity of the thorax, is very subject to inflammation. This may take place at any period of life, but it is more frequent at the age when the body is just arrived at the adult state, and all its actions are carried on with vigour, than either in childhood or in advanced age. The pleura appears to be more liable to inflammation than any membrane lining those cavities which have no external opening; as the peritonaeum, the tunica vaginalis testis, and some others. This may arise from the following causes: The branches of the intercostal vessels, which are very numerous, piercing through the substance of the intercostal muscles, communicate a good deal by anastomosis, with the external vessels on the sides of the chest. Hence whatever may act upon these external vessels so as to excite contraction in them, may be supposed capable of producing an accumulation of blood, as well as an increased action in the inner branches of the intercostals, many of which are distributed upon the pleura. Many of the inhabitants of this country, from their mode of dress, have their chests much exposed to the influence of a cold and very uncertain climate, and hence the blood is frequently thrown inwards into the small vessels ramifying upon the pleura. For these reasons probably the pleura is more liable to inflammation than other membranes investing cavities, which have no external opening. This is so much the case, that one can hardly examine the chest of any person who has arrived at the adult state, without perceiving more or less the traces of a present or former inflammation.

When the pleura is inflamed, it becomes thicker than it is naturally, and in some degree pulpy. There are also interspersed through it a great number of very small vessels containing florid blood, and a layer of coagulable lymph is at the same time thrown out upon its surface. This layer is sometimes very thin, and at other times of considerable thickness. It is either smooth upon its surface, or it throws out many small flocculi, which exhibit the appearance of a rich lace-work. A serous fluid is also poured into the cavity of the thorax, in which are floating many small broken laminae of the coagulable lymph; and there is occasionally some mixture of pus.

The coagulable lymph, covering the pleura which forms the external membrane of the lungs, frequently adheres to that which covers the pleura that is reflected on the inside of the parietes of the chest, either in small portions, or by extended surfaces. Upon such occasions I have sometimes been able to trace the gradual change of the adhesion, from the state of coagulable lymph to that of cellular membrane. This coagulable lymph may be shewn to be vascular by injection, as we have already mentioned in the inflammation of the pericardium. When the pleura is inflamed which covers the lungs, the substance of the latter is frequently inflamed to some depth.

Adhesions in the Cavity of the Thorax

Adhesions are often found between that portion of the pleura which covers the lungs, and that other portion of it which lines the ribs, the intercostal spaces, and the convex surface of the diaphragm, while there is no sign whatever of present inflammation. These adhesions are often partial, and they are most commonly to be found at the upper and posterior part of the chest; but they are sometimes extended over the whole cavity. They either connect the parts together closely, in which case they often consist of a firm thick membrane; or they connect them loosely, and then they consist of a soft spongy membrane, which exactly resembles the common cellular membrane of the body. Such adhesions are the consequence of inflammation, and are perhaps the most common morbid appearance to be found in dead bodies.

Empyema

Pus is not unfrequently accumulated in the cavity of the chest, forming the disease called empyema. This may either arise from the blood vessels of the pleura being in such a state of inflammation as to form pus, or from the bursting of some abscess in the lungs, so as to evacuate its pus into the cavity of the thorax. When pus is formed by an inflamed state of the pleura, there is no occasion for ulceration to take place. The pleura is found entire, but is covered with a layer of the coagulable lymph. This fact has been long ago ascertained by the late Dr. Hunter. The formation of the pus depends on a certain state of action in the vessels of the pleura, or more probably of the layer of the coagulable lymph which covers it. The pus may either occupy the whole of one of the cavities of the chest, or may be confined to a part of it by adhesions taking place between the lungs and the pleura, which invests the ribs and the intercostal spaces. When pus is evacuated into the cavity of the chest by the bursting of an abscess in the lungs, it is almost always confined within certain limits by adhesions. In cases of empyema, for the most part, there is not any particular appearance of the chest observable on the outside: there is sometimes however a fullness to be perceived externally on the side where the matter is accumulated, and even occasionally an evident swelling between two of the ribs, as of matter pointing. Ulceration has also been known to take place in one or more of the intercostal spaces, so that the matter has been evacuated externally. There is an example in Dr. Hunter's collection, where the matter had been evacuated from the chest by a good many openings in the intercostal spaces.

Hydrothorax

A watery fluid is not uncommonly found in one or both cavities of the chest, forming the disease called hydrothorax. It is often attended with the accumulation of water in other parts of the body, especially in the pericardium, and the cellular membrane of the lower extremities. The fluid in hydrothorax is commonly of a brown or yellowish colour, but occasionally has a reddish colour, arising from the mixture of the red globules of blood. It resembles in its properties the serum. It is found to vary a good deal in quantity in different cases, sometimes amounting only to a few ounces, and at other times to several quarts. When it is accumulated in very large quantity in either side of the chest, that side appears to be fuller to the eye externally; and when the cavity is laid open after death, the lungs on that side are found more or less compressed. I have seen a lung so compressed, as not to be larger than the closed fist.

Water is likewise found in the cavity of the chest where there are considerable adhesions. This shews that a good deal of inflammation had formerly taken place, which had probably, by throwing out a considerable quantity of serum, laid the foundation of the hydrothorax (16).

The Pleura almost dry

In opening into the cavity of the chest, there is commonly found a good deal of moisture upon the surface of the pleura. This is intended to lubricate the surface of the cavity of the chest, for the more easy motion of the lungs within it. Sometimes, however, I have seen the moisture in very small quantity, so that the pleura might almost be said to be dry. This was occasioned either by a deficiency in the action of the exhalant arteries of the pleura, or by an increased action of its absorbents.

Ossification of the Pleura

It sometimes happens, although I believe rarely, that a portion of the pleura is converted into bone. This consists of a thin plate and sometimes extends over a considerable surface of the pleura. In all the cases which I have seen, the bony matter seemed to me to be exactly like ordinary bone. I have never seen it form a thick irregular knob, but always a thin plate. The cause which first excites this deseased process is very difficult to determine; but there can be no doubt that the bone is formed by the small vessels of the pleura, which secrete bony matter from the blood. This process is not peculiar to the pleura, but takes place in almost every part of the body: I believe, however, that it is more common

16. This circumstance is illustrated in several instances by Mr. Cruikshank, in his Treatise upon the Absorbent System. See 2d edition, p. 116.

in the pleura, than in any other similar membrane. In the cases which I have observed, this process seemed not to have been attended with much inconvenience. There was no inflammation found in the pleura surrounding the bone, nor in the substance of the lungs under it. It is reasonable to think however, if the bone were to grow irregularly, so as to form sharp processes, that it might excite inflammation, and lay the foundation of a fatal disease (17).

SYMPTOMS

The symptoms which attend inflammation of the pleura are very well ascertained. There is more or less of symptomatic fever; an acute pain in some part of the chest, more commonly in the side, which is increased upon inspiration; a great difficulty in lying upon the diseased side; difficult respiration; a cough, which at first is dry, but is afterwards accompanied with a secretion and expectoration of mucus from the inner membrane of the trachea and its branches.

There would often seem to be slight degrees of inflammation in the pleura, where the symptoms above stated do not exist at all, or are so obscurely marked as to be altogether overlooked. In examining the chest of adults after death, it rarely happens that adhesions are not discovered in some part of it, uniting the surface of the lungs to the pleura which lines the parietes of the chest. The marked symptoms of pleurisy, however, are by no means so frequent. It seems, therefore, probable, that slight inflammations may attack the pleura, sufficient however to throw out coagulable lymph, which is afterwards changed into adhesions, and yet that persons thus affected shall not be sensible of any disease in the chest. If this supposition be not granted, then coagulable lymph may be thrown out upon the surface of the pleura, and adhesions be formed without inflammation. This conjecture is not so probable as the other.

Where adhesions in the chest are long, so as not to impede the

---

17. A case is mentioned by Dr. Soemmerring, where a part of the lungs was found inflamed and suppurated under an ossification of the pleura. See Soemmerring, Germ. Translat. of the Morbid Anatomy, p. 43.

free motion of the lungs, respiration is not sensibly affected by them. But where the adhesions are short, tying as it were the lungs closely to the parietes of the chest, and more especially if they be extended over every part of the cavity, then respiration is difficult and accompanied with a cough, but there are no symptoms of fever.

Empyema may be distinguished with a good deal of certainty, after inflammation of the pleura or of the lungs, by rigors having taken place, by a remission of the pain, by the cough and difficulty of breathing continuing, and by the person being able to lie more easily upon the diseased side than the other. There is sometimes a very evident, enlargement of the side where the matter is accumulated.

When water is accumulated in the chest, it can generally be sufficiently distinguished in practice by the following symptoms.

There is great difficulty of breathing, and the patient cannot rest in bed unless the head and the upper part of the trunk be more or less elevated from the horizontal posture. The sleep is often suddenly interrupted by alarms and disagreeable dreams; the urine is in very small quantity, and there is commonly anasarca of the legs. The pulse is generally, but not always, irregular. There is a paleness in the countenance, with a purple hue of the lips and of the cheeks, if the latter should happen to have any tinge remaining. This effect is produced by the lungs being incapable of sufficiently expanding themselves to receive the quantity of air which is necessary for giving the usual florid colour to the blood in the branches of the pulmonary artery.

When ossification of the pleura is of small extent, respiration cannot be affected by it; but when it is large it must produce difficulty of breathing, either by preventing the full expansion of the lungs, or the free motion of the ribs, according to its situation: Some instances are known of respiration being injured from this cause.

Where the ossification has produced inflammation of the pleura and lungs, symptoms of inflammation will take place as above described, but probably in some cases there may be peculiar symptoms, depending chiefly on the different irritability of different constitutions. In one case there were paroxisms of convulsive difficulty of breathing, palpitation of the heart, a quick irregular pulse, and a distressing sense of instant suffocation (18).

18. See Mr. Weldon's Observations in Surgery, p. 75 and 76.

CHAPTER IV

DISEASED APPEARANCES OF THE LUNGS

Inflammation

INFLAMMATION of the substance of the lungs, I believe, seldom takes place without some similar affection of the pleura; at least in the instances which I have seen, this has been most frequently the case. When a portion of the lungs is inflamed, its spongy structure appears much redder than usual, the colour being chiefly florid but partly of a darker hue. This arises from a much greater number of small vessels than usual, being distributed upon the cells of the lungs, which are capable of admitting the red globules of the blood. There is also an extravasation of the coagulable lymph into the substance of the lungs, and sometimes of blood. The extravasated blood has been said upon some occasions to be in very large quantity; but this has never fallen under my own observations.

That portion of the lungs which is inflamed becomes considerably heavier than in the natural state, from the accumulation of blood in its vessels, and the extravasation of the coagulable lymph; it therefore commonly sinks in water. It feels like a solid substance when pressed by the fingers, and there is no crackling of air as in the healthy structure. This however will be more or less marked, according to the degree of the inflammation.

The pleura covering the inflamed portion of the lungs is also commonly affected with inflammation; it is crowded with fine red vessels, and has generally lying upon it a layer of coagulable lymph.

This inflamed state of the lungs is to be distinguished from blood accumulated in some part of them after death in consequence of gravitation. From the body lying in the horizontal posture after death, blood is often accumulated at the posterior part of the lungs, giving them there a deeper colour, and rendering them heavier. In this case there will be found no crowd of fine vessels filled with blood, nor any other mark of inflammation of the pleura. Where blood too is accumulated in any part of a lung after death, from gravitation, it is always of a dark colour; but where blood is accumulated from inflammation, the inflamed part will appear, in a great measure, florid.

Abscesses

It is very common to find abscesses in the lungs. These sometimes consist of small cavities containing pus and at other times the cavities are very large so that the greater part of the substance of the lungs has been destroyed. These cavities sometimes communicate only with branches of the trachea, which are destroyed in the progress of the ulceration; at other times they open into the cavity of the chest, emptying their contents there, and forming the disease which is called empyema. When abscesses are deeply seated in the substance of the lungs, the pleura is commonly not affected; but when abscesses are formed near the surface, it is almost constantly inflamed. The lungs round the boundaries of an abscess, when it has arisen from common inflammation, are more solid in their texture, in consequence of coagulable lymphs being thrown out during the progress of the inflammation. When the abscesses are scrofulous, the texture of the lungs in the neighbourhood is sometimes not firmer than usual, but presents the common natural appearance. This I believe to be principally the case when the abscesses are small, and placed at a considerable distance from each other. When a portion of the lungs is crowded with tubercles, and some of these are converted into abscesses, the intermediate substance of the lungs is often of a very solid texture. When blood vessels are traced into an abscess of the lungs, I have found them, upon examination, very much contracted, just before they reach the abscess, so that the opening of their extremities has been closed up entirely. On such occasion it will require a probe to be pushed with a good deal of force, in order to open again their extremities. In these contracted vessels the blood is coagulated, as it is under similar circumstances in other parts of the body (19). This change in the blood vessels is, no doubt, with a view to prevent large haemorrhages from taking place, which would certainly be almost immediately fatal.

Tubercles

There is no morbid appearance so common in the lungs as that of tubercles. These consist of rounded firm white bodies, interspersed through their substance. They are probably formed in the cellular structure, which connects the air cells of the lungs together, and are not a morbid affection of glands, as has been frequently imagined. There is no glandular structure in the cellular connecting membrane of the lungs; and on the inside of the branches of the trachea, where there are follicles, tubercles have never been seen. They are at first very small, being not larger than the heads of very small pins, and in this case are frequently accumulated in small clusters. The smaller tubercles of a cluster probably grow together and form one larger tubercle. The most ordinary size of tubercles is about that of a garden pea, but they are subject in this respect to much variety. They adhere pretty closely to the substance of the lungs, have no peculiar covering or capsule, and have little or no vascularity. When cut into, they are found to consist of a white, smooth substance, having a firm texture, and often contain in part a thick curdly pus. When a tubercle is almost entirely changed into pus, it appears like a white capsule, in which the pus is lodged. When several tubercles of considerable size are grown together, so as to form a pretty large tuberculated mass, pus is very generally found upon cutting into it. The pus is frequently thick and curdly; but when in considerable quantity, it is thinner, and resembles very much the pus from a common sore. In cutting into the substance of the lungs, a number of abscesses is sometimes found, from pretty large tubercles having advanced from a state of suppuration. In the interstices between these tubercles, the lungs are frequently of a harder, firmer texture, with the cells in a great measure obliterated. The texture of the lungs on many occasions, however, round

19. See Dr. Stark's works, p. 28.

the boundaries of an abscess, is perfectly natural.

I have sometimes seen a number of small abscesses interspersed through the lungs, each of which was not larger than a pea. The pus in these is rather thicker than what arises from common inflammation, and resembles scrofulous pus. It is probable that these abscesses have been produced by a number of small scattered tubercles taking on the process of suppuration. The lungs immediately surrounding these abscesses are often of a perfectly healthy structure, none of the cells being closed up by adhesions.

When tubercles are converted into abscesses, pthisis pulmonalis is produced, one of the most destructive diseases in this island. Tubercles are sometimes found in the lungs of children at a very early age, viz. two or three years old; but they most frequently occur shortly before the completion of the growth. They are apt, likewise, to be formed at rather an advanced age.

In cutting into the lungs, a considerable portion of their structure sometimes appears to be changed into a whitish soft matter, somewhat intermediate between a solid and a fluid, like a scrofulous gland just beginning to suppurate. This appearance I believe is produced by scrofulous matter being deposited in the cellular substance of a certain portion of the lungs, and advancing towards suppuration. It seems to be the same matter with that of the tubercle, but only diffused uniformly over a considerable portion of the lungs, while the tubercle is circumscribed.

Soft pulpy Tubercle

I have seen another sort of tubercle in the lungs, which I believe to be very rare. It consists of a soft tumour, formed of a light brown, smooth substance. This is not contained in any proper capsule, but adheres immediately to the common structure of the lungs. In cutting through several of these tumours I did not find any of them in a state of suppuration. They were commonly as large as a goosberry, and were chiefly placed upon the surface of the lungs; some, however, were scattered through their substance, of a smaller size. These are very different in their appearance from the common tubercle last described.

Water accumulated in the substance of the lungs

The structure of the lungs may be said to consist of air cells, and the common cellular membrane of the body. In this cellular membrane there is always some moisture, which is necessary for the easy motion of one part of the lungs upon another in their contraction and dilatation. There is a considerable difference in the quantity of this moisture in different persons, as may be seen by cutting into the substance of the lungs; for under such circumstances there will always ooze out from the cut surface more or less of an aqueous fluid mixed with globules of air. Sometimes, however, the quantity is so large that it amounts to a disease, forming what may be called anasarca of the lungs. It has not occurred to me to see any well marked example of this disease, but it has been observed by others (20). It is hardly necessary to mention, that in proportion to the accumulation of the water the air cells must be necessarily compressed, so that a sufficient quantity of air cannot be admitted into the lungs for producing the due degree of influence upon the blood.

Lungs distended with Air

In opening into the chest, it is not unusual, to find that the lungs do not collapse, but that they fill up the cavity completely on each side of the heart. When examined, their cells appear full of air, so that a prodigious number of small white vesicles are seen upon the surface of the lungs immediately under the pleura. The branches of the trachea are often at the same time a good deal filled with a mucous fluid.

Air Cells of the Lungs enlarged

The lungs are sometimes, although I believe very rarely, formed into pretty large cells, so as to resemble somewhat the lungs of an amphibious animal. Of this I have now seen three instances. The

---

20. See Dr. Soemmerring's German Translation of the Morbid Anatomy, p. 45.

enlargement of the cells cannot well be supposed to arise from any other cause, than the air being not allowed the common free egress from the lungs, and therefore accumulating in them. It is not improbable also, that this accumulation may sometimes break down two or three contiguous cells into one, and thereby form a cell of a very large size.

Air Vesicles attached to the Edge of the Lungs

Vesicles containing air have occasionally been seen attached to the edge of the lungs. They do not communicate, however, with the structure of this organ, but are complete in themselves. Upon the first view, it might be thought probable that they were merely some of the air cells enlarged; but as they do not communicate with any of the air cells, this opinion is not well founded. It is most likely that they are a morbid structure, formed in the same manner as the air vesicles attached to the intestines and mesentery of some quadrupeds, and that the very minute blood vessels which ramify upon the vesicles, have the power of secreting the air (21).

Lungs changed into a substance like Liver

The lungs are sometimes converted into a solid substance very much resembling the liver. It has nearly the same solidity, and the same general appearance. I have only seen an example of this change in a preparation, and I am inclined to believe that it had been produced by a wide extended inflammation, in which a large quantity of coagulable lymph had been extravasated into the substance of the lungs. The extravasation would necessarily render the texture of the lungs very solid; and the history of the symptoms which have been observed to attend similar morbid changes, supports this opinion. The symptoms are those which are produced by an inflammation of the lungs.

Lungs converted into Bone

Part of the lungs is occasionally converted into bony substance;

---

21. See Hunter's Animal Economy, p. 165.

but this is a very rare disease. The small vessels ramifying through the substance of the lungs under such circumstances separate bony matter from the blood. In the only instance which I have known of this complaint, the process would appear to have been rapid. There was great difficulty of breathing before the person died, but this difficulty had been only for a very few weeks. Each of the lungs was undergoing the same change of structure which had made considerable progress. In the particular case to which I allude, there had been a very strong disposition to form bone in the constitution. A very large bony tumour had been formed round one of the knees of this person; and very soon after the knee and leg were removed by amputation, the difficulty of breathing began, which was occasioned by a part of the lungs being converted into bone. In this case there was a transference of the disease from an external to an internal part, similar to the translation of gout or rheumatism.

A solid Tumour compressing the Lungs

I have also seen a tumour as large as an orange, attached to the lungs on one side by a loose membranous connection and in some degree compressing them; this tumour consisted of a porous substance, which resembled neither the structure of what is commonly understood to be a scirrhous nor that of a scrofulous tumour, but had an appearance somewhat peculiar to itself.

Earthy Concretions in the Lungs

Earthy concretions have occasionally been found in the lungs, although it is a rare appearance of disease. These are often small, but sometimes form masses of a considerable size (22). Even a considerable portion of the lungs has been known to be changed into an earthy substance (23).

Hydatids

Hydatids are also sometimes formed in the lungs, and are many

22. Vid. Morgagni, Epist. XVII. Art. 19. XV. Art. 25.
23. Vid. Morgagni, Epist. XXII. Art. 15.

of them brought up by coughing. They are of the same sort with the hydatids formed in the liver, the nature of which we shall endeavor to explain afterwards.

SYMPTOMS

In inflammation of the substance of the lungs, the symptoms correspond a good deal with those of pleurisy. Indeed inflammation of the lungs is almost constantly attended with inflammation of the pleura, so that it is difficult to discriminate between them in practice. But it is of little consequence to be able to do this, as a means of cure are the same in both diseases. When the inflammation of the lungs is pure, the pleura being not affected, the pain in the chest has been observed to be more obtuse than in pleurisy, and the pulse to be less hard. The respiration is very difficult, and the veins of the neck are sometimes observed to be distended with blood, the face to be tumid, and there is a purplish hue of the lips and cheeks. These effects arise from the venal blood being transmitted with difficulty through the inflamed lungs. This is occasionally by an extravasation of the coagulable lymph into a considerable part of their substance, which both prevents the lungs from sufficiently expanding themselves, and compresses many air cells, so that the proper quantity of air is not admitted into the lungs for producing the full change of colour upon the blood.

When inflammation of the lungs terminates in suppuration, it may be known by rigors, by a diminution of the pain in the chest, and by an expectoration of pus.

When tubercles are forming in the lungs, but have not advanced to suppuration, they are attended with a slight cough, with occasional difficulty of breathing, and a pulse somewhat accelerated. These are symptoms which commonly usher in phthisis pulmonalis and are frequently overlooked, both by the patients themselves and their friends. When the tubercles have begun to suppurate, and abscesses to be formed, then there is an expectoration of a thick pus, which is occasionally tinged with blood, emaciation, debility, and that peculiar affection of the system which is known by the name of hectic fever.

The symptoms attending the large brown tubercle are unknown to me.

When the cells of the lungs are much enlarged in their size, persons have been remarked to be long subject to difficulty of breathing; but I believe no symptom is at present known, by which this disease may be discriminated from some others incident to the chest.

In some cases in which the lungs have been converted into a substance like the liver, symptoms have been observed similar to those which attend inflammation of the lungs. I am inclined to believe that this appearance of the lungs is produced by an extensive extravasation of coagulable lymph into their substance, during an attack of inflammation.

When earthy concretions are formed in the lungs, persons are more or less subject to difficulty of breathing and a cough. Occasionally some of these concretions are coughed up, which circumstance becomes the discriminating mark of this disease. Without it, this disease could not be distinguished from several others which attack the chest.

When hydatids are formed in the lungs, they produce a cough, difficulty of breathing, and some frequency of the pulse. They are occasionally forced up by a violent fit of coughing; and this circumstance only can discriminate the disease in the living body.

CHAPTER V

DISEASED APPEARANCES OF THE THYROID GLAND, THE LARYNX, AND THE PARTS CONTAINED IN THE POSTERIOR MEDIASTINUM

BEFORE we describe the diseased appearances of the parts which are contained in the posterior mediastinum, we shall take notice of the morbid changes to which the thyroid gland and the larynx are liable. These are so closely connected with the trachea, that a description of their morbid changes could not be introduced so properly in any other place.

Inflammation of the Thyroid Gland

The thyroid gland is sometimes attacked with common inflammation, but this happens rarely. There are no peculiar causes acting upon it to produce inflammation, and it would seem to be as little liable to be excited to this diseased action as any gland in the body. When the thyroid gland is inflamed, it exhibits the common appearances which take place in the inflammation of the substance of other parts. Its blood vessels are enlarged in their size, and the number of branches which are capable of containing the red globules of blood is increased. Hence it appears much more vascular than in a natural state. It is increased in its bulk, and feels considerably firmer to the touch than when healthy; and these effects are produced partly by the increased quantity of blood which is circulating through it, and partly by the extravasation of coagulable lymph, and perhaps of blood, into its substance.

Bronchocele

The morbid change of structure to which the thyroid gland is most liable, is that swelling of it called bronchocele. This is apt to take place in different individuals of the same family, and women are more liable to be affected with it than men. It is more prevalent in some districts of countries than in others, and those where it is most prevalent are mountainous.

The swelling of the thyroid gland in bronchocele often increases to a very large size, and sometimes grows irregularly, forming projecting tumours upon the anterior part of the neck. This irregularity of growth is more common in that part of Savoy, where the disease is endemial, than in Great Britain.

When a section is made of the thyroid gland affected with this disease, it is found to consist of a number of cells which contain a transparent viscid fluid. These cells vary in their size in different parts of the same gland, and in different swellings of the same kind in different individuals. Some of them are so large as to be able to contain a small pea, but most of them are of a smaller size. The viscid fluid, when the gland has been preserved for some time in spirits, is changed into a transparent jelly. From this account of the morbid change of structure which takes place in bronchocele, it seems not unreasonable to suppose that the swelling depends upon a vitiated and increased secretion in the gland. The secretion being in large quantity, gradually distends the cells, increasing thereby their capacity, and this enlargement of the cells forms the general swelling of the gland. What is now said, however, is thrown out merely as a conjecture, and should be received with caution.

Scirrhous of the Thyroid Gland

The thyroid gland sometimes becomes scirrhous, but is not so liable to this disease as some other glands of the body. When it is affected by this disease, it becomes enlarged in its size, but not to any considerable degree, and is hard to the feeling. When a section is made of it, it is found to consist of a solid substance, with very little of that cellular structure which is so strongly marked in bronchocele.

This gland is apt to become swelled and hard when ulcers are formed at the upper end of the oesophagus. This effect is sometimes produced by the ulcer of the oesophagus spreading to the thyroid gland. The same change, however, has been observed to take place where the ulcer had not reached so far, and where the gland was entire. This might lead to the opinion, that some ducts of communication exist between the thyroid gland and the upper part of the oesophagus. These ducts have been supposed by several anatomists, but their existence has never yet been demonstrated.

The Thyroid Gland converted into Bone

The thyroid gland, or a part of it, is occasionally changed in old people into a bony mass, but this disease is of rare occurrence. It is commonly, I believe, a disease of no consequence; but it is reasonable to think, that the bony mass by an irregular growth might in some instances so irritate the larynx, or the upper part of the trachea, as to produce inflammation and ulceration of these parts, and to prove ultimately fatal.

Larynx–The cartilages of the Larynx converted into Bone

The cartilages of the larynx sometimes become bony, either at the middle or a more advanced period of life. When the disposition to form bony matter in the larynx is not very strong, portions of the thyroid cartilage only are converted into bone; but when the disposition is powerful, then all the cartilages are changed into a bony substance. When this is the case they become liable to any changes which might take place in ordinary bone. Accordingly, some of these cartilages so changed into bone have been known to exfoliate, and to be thrown out by a violent fit of coughing or vomiting. Dr. Hunter had an opportunity of knowing an instance where the cricoid cartilage, being converted into bone, was separated by exfoliation, and afterwards coughed up. It is not to be understood from what has been said, that the cartilages of the larynx, when changed into bone, are more liable to become dead and exfoliate than the common bones of the body. The instances in which they have been known to exfoliate are, I believe, extremely rare.

Ulcers in the cavity of the Larynx

The inner membrane of the larynx is very apt to be inflamed, and this generally accompanies the inflammation of the inner membrane of the trachea, as we shall have occasion to mention afterwards. Sometimes, however, an inflammation shall take place which is confined to the cavity of the larynx, and it shall occasionally advance to suppuration. Of this I have known several instances. Suppuration is most apt to take place in the sacculi laryngis: and the ulcers which I have seen there are sometimes attended with a scrofulous thickening of the surrounding parts.

Diseased Appearances of the Parts contained in the Posterior Mediastinum

By the posterior mediastinum, is meant that space which lies between the laminae of the pleura, that pass from the root of the lungs to each side of the spine. The space is of considerable size, and contains a portion of the trachea arteria, of the oesophagus, of the thoracic duct, of the descending aorta, and the vena azygos, besides some absorbent glands.

Diseased Appearances of the Trachea

The inner membrane of the trachea is not uncommonly inflamed to a greater or less degree. In this state it is crowded with minute florid vessels, which give it a general appearance of vascularity. When there is no inflammation, it appears in the dead body a white pulpy membrane, and there are rarely to be seen any red vessels ramifying in it. While the inner membrane is inflamed, the secretion from its glands is very much increased, and therefore its cavity is found a good deal filled with a mucous fluid; even pus is sometimes formed, and both fluids are mixed with globules of air. This is the state of the trachea in a very violent catarrh, and also in some cases where there are scrofulous abscesses of the lungs attended with hoarseness, and a sense of soreness along the trachea: the same appearances are also observable in the inner membrane of the larynx.

Appearances of the Trachea in the Croup

When the inner membrane of the trachea is inflamed, it is sometimes lined with a layer of a yellowish pulpy matter. This does not adhere firmly to the inner membrane, but may be easily separated. It extends from the upper part of the cavity of the larynx, into the small branches of the trachea, which are distributed through the substance of the lungs. There is at the same time a good deal of mucus in the trachea and its branches, together with a mixture of pus. This is the appearance of the inside of the trachea, in patients who have died from the croup.

Polypus

The trachea and its branches are sometimes lined with a layer of a yellowish or whitish matter, forming a sort of tube, which is applied to the inner surface loosely. It has not occurred to me to see any instance of it in the dead bodies which I have examined; but I have seen several examples of it in preparations. The inner membrane of the trachea seems to be perfectly natural, and the layer of adventitious membrane resembles exactly the coagulable lymph which is thrown out in any parts of the body; I have therefore no doubt of its being that substance. Since this disease (which is called polypus) lasts for a long time, and is not attended with symptoms of inflammation, it appears probable that the vessels of the inner membrane of the trachea possess a power of separating the coagulable lymph from the blood, and that this disease consists in a peculiar action of these vessels.

The trachea is sometimes filled with a solid substance, of the same kind with what we have described. Of this I have only seen one instance, and it occurs, I believe, much more rarely than the other.

The tubular substances which are thrown out from the trachea in coughing, and which constitute the most ordinary form of polypus, were considered formerly, by some anatomists of distinguished reputation, as blood vessels. It is singular that they should have paid so little attention to the appearance of these tubular substances as to have mistaken them for blood vessels; and it is still more singular, that it should never have occurred to their reflection, that blood vessels of such a size could not be coughed up, without a very large quantity of blood passing along with them.

A more modern opinion about the nature of these tubular substances has been that they consist of dried mucus This, although more plausible than the former, is equally ill founded. The mucus which is secreted by the inner membrane of the trachea, is exactly of the same kind with that secreted by the inner membrane of the nose. Every person is acquainted with the appearance of the mucus of the nose when dried. The mucus of the trachea, when dried would have the same appearance. The tubular substances coughed up in polypus of the trachea, present an appearance to the eye very different, and (as has been already noticed) look exactly like the coagulable lymph. The influence of the air in drying the mucus would seem to extend but a little way from the external surface of the body, for the mucus is fluid even in the posterior nostrils.

Trachea scirrhous

The trachea I have seen narrowed in diameter for two or three inches, thickened in its substance, and the inner membrane has been raised into a number of little hard tubercles. This state of the trachea was accompanied with a scirrhous affection of some absorbent glands, which closely adhered to it; and it appeared to me that the disease in the glands has spread so as to affect the trachea.

Rings of the Trachea ossified

The cartilaginous rings of the Trachea occasionally become ossified. When the ossification is inconsiderable, the function of the trachea will hardly be affected by it; but where the rings are entirely ossified, the flexibility of the trachea must be much lessened, and its cavity will not admit of being so much contracted as in the healthy state, by the action of muscular fibres, which form a part of its structure. In consequence of this the mucus which is occasionally accumulated will not be so readily expelled by coughing, and probably the air will not be thrown out in so small a column, nor with so much momentum.

Ulcers of the Trachea

The trachea is doubtless liable to be destroyed in part by ulceration, from causes acting immediately upon itself; but in the instances which I have seen, the ulceration has been connected with ulceration of the oesophagus. As the oesophagus is more liable to this disease, it is probable that in such cases the ulceration has begun in the oesophagus, and spread to the trachea.

Diseased Appearances of the Oesophagus

The oesophagus is frequently lined with a layer of the coagulable lymph, which is continued from the cavity of the mouth.

This, it is said, sometimes extends over the whole intestinal canal; but I believe this appearance to be extremely rare, and it commonly terminates at the lower end of the oesophagus. The inner membrane of the mouth is much more vascular than in its natural state, shewing a deep red colour; but in examinations after death the appearance of greater redness is sometimes scarcely observable in the oesophagus. This disease is known under the name of aphthae, and is much more often to be observed in the living than the dead body.

Spasmodic stricture of the Oesophagus

The oesophagus is liable to stricture, produced by the contraction of its muscular fibres at some particular part. This disease is most common in women whose constitutions are delicate, and much subject to nervous influence. When such a disease is examined in the dead body, the oesophagus is found to be more or less contracted in some part of it, and it feels harder than usual, as happens to all muscles in a contracted state. There is no appearance of diseased structure usually combined with it. I can suppose, however, that this contraction might lay the foundation of a permanent, and even a fatal disease. The muscular fibres of the oesophagus might so press on the inner membrane, as to excite inflammation in it, which might advance to suppuration, and would most probably terminate fatally.

Stricture from the puckering of the inner Membrane of the Oesophagus

I once saw a very unusual stricture of the oesophagus. It consisted in its inner membrane being puckered together, so as to form a narrowness of the canal at a particular part, which would hardly allow a common garden pea to pass. There was no appearance, however, of diseased structure in the inner membrane which was so contracted, and the muscular part of the oesophagus surrounding it was perfectly sound. I know that this disease was very slow in its progress, for the person in whom it took place had been for many years affected with a difficulty of swallowing, and could only swallow substances of an extremely small size.

Stricture attended with Ulcer

The most common appearance of disease in the oesophagus, is that of an ulcer in its cavity. Ulcers of the oesophagus are sometimes of a common nature, but most frequently they are attended with a scirrhous affection. When they arise from common inflammation, the structure of the oesophagus immediately surrounding the ulcer is but little thickened, and there is the appearance of the usual erosion in ulcers. When the ulcer is of a scirrhous nature the oesophagus in the neighbourhood is very much thickened, and is very hard in its texture. When this texture is examined, it either consists of a hard, uniformly fleshy substance, or this is a little intersected by membranes, or it is gristly. Under such circumstances, the canal of the oesophagus is always more or less narrowed, and in some cases is almost wholly obliterated. It is worthy of remark, that these ulcers happen most frequently, either immediately under the pharynx, or near the cardia.

Any substance capable of irritating the inner membrane of the oesophagus, by having sharp hard projections, will doubtless be more likely to affect the oesophagus, where it first enters into it. In an oesophagus, therefore, predisposed to scirrhous, such an accident may prove an exciting cause, and the disease will more frequently take place at its upper end. At the cardia too, there is a peculiar arrangement of the muscular fibres, which are capable of acting in some degree like a sphincter, and which probably produce on many occasions a narrowness of the canal there. This will render the oesophagus at the cardia more liable to be injured by the passage of any hard substance, and may ultimately lay the foundation of a scirrhous ulcer. This is the account which the late Dr. Hunter used to give of the frequent situation of ulcers at the upper and lower extremities of the oesophagus, and it seems to have great weight. It happens however, most commonly that ulcers of the oesophagus arise spontaneously, or in other words, from causes within itself which we cannot ascertain. When an ulcer takes place at the upper end of the oesophagus, it is apt to spread into the substance of the thyroid gland. In this case the gland becomes hard, enlarged, and ulcerated: but in some instances it has been known to enlarge, where the ulcer of the oesophagus had not spread so far as to reach it.

Oesophagus cartilaginous

A portion of the oesophagus has been observed by some anatomists to be converted into cartilage, and to have its diameter at that part very much diminished in size (24). This was probably only a strong example of the gristly texture above described.

Fungus in the Pharynx

I have seen an instance of a fungus arising on the inside of the pharynx and the upper end of the oesophagus, which is to be considered as a rare disease. When cut into it appeared to have a fibrous structure, disposed in some measure at right angles to the

24. Vid. Bonet, Tom. II. p. 32.

inner membrane upon which it was formed, and was ulcerated on its surface.

Scrofulous swelling in the Pharynx

It has occurred to me likewise to see a scrofulous swelling at the lower end of the pharynx and the beginning of the oesophagus. When cut into it appeared to consist of the same kind of matter as a scrofulous absorbent gland. It grew upon that side of the pharynx which is next to the larynx, and the patient for this reason had not only lost almost entirely the power of swallowing but was not able to speak except in the smallest whisper.

Pouch formed at the lower end of the Pharynx

The pharynx, at its lower extremity, has been known to be dilated into a pouch of a considerable size, which passed behind the oesophagus. This may be supposed to be very rare, but there is an instance of it preserved in Dr. Hunter's collection. The pouch in this case began to be formed in consequence of a cherry-stone having rested there for some time, which had made a kind of bed for itself. It remained in that situation for three days, and then was brought up by a violent fit of coughing. A part of the food always rested afterwards in the cavity made by the cherry-stone, by which it was gradually enlarged. At length, in the course of about five years, the cavity was enlarged into a bag of considerable size, sufficient to contain several ounces of fluid. This bag passed down a good way behind the oesophagus, and the oesophagus necessarily acquired a valvular communication with it. In proportion as the bag enlarged, this valvular communication would become more and more complete, till at length every kind of food must have rested in the bag, and could not pass into the oesophagus. In this way the person was destroyed. The lower end of the pharynx, is, perhaps, the only part of the canal where such an accident can happen. The pharynx is not contracted gradually, so as to lose itself insensibly in the oesophagus, but contracts itself rather suddenly at the lower end. Hence a little recess is formed, in which an extraneous body may occasionally rest. This would be most apt to happen at the posterior part; so that if the recess should be enlarged into a cavity, it would generally pass behind the oesophagus. The particulars of this singular case have been published in the Medical observations (25).

The descending Aorta

There is hardly any other disease of the descending aorta within the posterior mediastinum, than aneurysm. This consists in the aorta being a good deal enlarged beyond its natural size, in its coats being irregularly thickened, and more readily divisible into layers than in a healthy state. Little thin laminae of bony matter are also frequently deposited behind the inner membrane. This appearance of disease, has been formerly explained more particularly. It is rare that this part of the aorta becomes aneurysmal, unless there be a general aneurysmal affection over the arterial system.

The Vena Azygos varicose

The vena azygos is very seldom diseased. I have seen it, however, varicose, and very much enlarged. This change in it took place from particular circumstances. A considerable portion of the vena cava inferior had become obliterated; in consequence of this, the usual vena azygos, together with an uncommon one on the left side, were the only channels through which the blood could return by a circuitous route to the heart; they were therefore necessarily, from the impetus of the blood, much enlarged in size, and for the same reason likewise varicose. This case I have more particularly described in the Medical and Chirurgical Transactions (26).

Vena Azygos ruptured

The vena azygos has been known to be ruptured, when very much distended with blood (27). Such a case has not come under my own observation, and I believe it to be very uncommon.

---

25. See the Medical Observations, Vol. III. p. 85.
26. See p. 125, &c. Vol. I.
27. Vid. Morgagni, Epist. XXVI. Art. 29.

The Thoracic duct varicose

The thoracic duct also is subject to very few diseases. I have never seen any other except that of its being very much enlarged and varicose.

In the instance to which I allude, it was very nearly as large as the usual size of a subclavian vein, but nothing could be detected in the neighbouring parts, capable of accounting for this appearance. There was no obstruction at the entrance of the thoracic duct into the venal system, which might naturally have been expected. This diseased appearance of the thoracic duct has already been taken notice of by Mr. Cruikshank in his treatise on the Absorbent System (28).

Thoracic Duct obstructed

The thoracic duct has been known to be obstructed by an earthy matter deposited in its cavity (29). It does not necessarily happen when the thoracic duct is at some part obstructed, that chyle is prevented from entering into the system of blood vessels. The thoracic duct sometimes sends off one or more considerable branches, which unite again with the principal trunk. If under such circumstances an obstruction should take place in a part of the principal trunk, between the origin and the termination of those branches, no bad effect would follow; one or more of these branches would become enlarged, and convey the chyle in its full quantity to the blood.

Thoracic Duct ruptured

The thoracic duct has also been known to be ruptured; although this is exceedingly rare.

Absorbent Glands scrofulous

The absorbent glands in the posterior mediastinum, as well as in every other part of the body, are liable to several diseases. The

28. See second edition, p. 207; and it is represented in an engraving, Plate V.
29. Vid. Lieutaud, Tom. II. p. 93.

most common morbid affection is scrofula. In this case they are frequently a good deal enlarged, and feel somewhat softer to the touch than in their healthy structure. When cut into, however, they sometimes exhibit very much the natural appearance; but it is more common to find that some of them contain a white, soft cheesy matter, mixed with a thick pus: this is the most decided mark of scrofulous affection. When the absorbent glands in this situation are very much enlarged, they necessarily produce some difficulty of breathing, both by pressing on the lungs and the trachea. They may occasion also some difficulty of swallowing.

Absorbent Glands scirrhous

I have seen the absorbent glands in the neighbourhood of the trachea affected with scirrhous, although it is a rare disease in them. They were much enlarged and very hard to the touch. When cut into they exhibited a harder texture, somewhat intersected by membrane, so as to resemble what is called scirrhous in other parts of the body. The trachea in contact with these glands was also affected. In this case the thyroid gland was scirrhous, and it is probable that the disease spread from the thyroid to the absorbent glands, and so to the trachea.

Absorbent Glands bony

The absorbent glands near the trachea are sometimes converted into a bony or earthy matter; and I think that this disease is more common in the absorbent glands at the root of the trachea, than in any other part of the body. These glands when so diseased, by pressing against the trachea or oesophagus, occasionally produce ulcers in them.

The Anterior Mediastinum

By the anterior mediastinum is meant the space inclosed between the laminae of the pleura, which pass from the sternum to the pericardium; it contains little else than cellular membrane, with perhaps a small portion of fat; and in the younger subject the thymus gland.

It is seldom found with any diseased appearance in it. Abscesses are occasionally formed there, but rarely. Water too is sometimes found in the cells of its cellular membrane. I have also seen air accumulated in these cells.

Fat is occasionally deposited in the mediastinum in considerable quantity. When the quantity is very large, it has been known to disturb the functions both of the heart and lungs.

Diseased Appearances of the Thymus Gland

The thymus gland is subject to few diseases, and is only of temporary existence; few instances therefore of morbid structure have been observed in it.

It would seem to be very little disposed to common inflammation; therefore abscesses have occurred in it very rarely, and have been but little noticed by authors.

It is more liable to be enlarged in its size, and to become hard in its texture. It once occurred to myself to observe an instance of this sort, but I had not an opportunity of examining it very minutely.

Small calculi have been said to be occasionally formed in the thymus gland (30).

SYMPTOMS

Inflammation of the thyroid gland may be known by an increase of its size and firmness, by a pain felt in it which is increased upon pressure, and which is probably also increased during the act of swallowing. It may be distinguished from some other swellings of this gland, as for instance from bronchocele, by its rapid progress, by the feeling of pain, and by its not increasing to a very large size.

It is worth while to remark, that practitioners ought to be particularly cautious to prevent inflammation of the thyroid gland from advancing to suppuration. If it should suppurate, and the pus

30. See Dr. Soemmerring's German Translation, p. 61.

be evacuated externally, there will be a scar in the neck; and if it should point internally, it will probably make its way into the cavity of the larynx or the trachea, and suffocate the patient. There is a preparation in Dr. Hunter's collection, shewing this fatal termination of inflammation in the thyroid gland. Every means should be attempted to make the inflammation terminate in resolution. When inflammation of the substance of any part terminates in resolution, the blood vessels gradually return to their natural mode of action, and their natural size: the deep seated absorbents are at the same time excited to an increased exertion, so as to remove the blood and the coagulable lymph which had been extravasated during the inflammation. This is one of the chief uses of the absorbent vessels which are distributed through the substance of parts (31).

Bronchocele may be distinguished from other swellings of the thyroid gland, by its slow growth, by the size at which it is capable of arriving, by its want of pain, by its commonly occurring at an early period of life, by the sensation it yields to the touch, which is that of more or less firmness, but not of great hardness, and by the health being unaffected by it.

Scirrhous of the thyroid gland may be distinguished from other swellings of it, by its great hardness, by occasional darting pains in the gland, and by this affection being most apt to occur in persons of an advanced age. The swelling likewise in scirrhous of the thyroid gland is seldom so large as in bronchocele.

Ossification in the thryoid gland can only be ascertained by an accurate examination of the part affected. If the ossification be upon the surface of the gland, the bony matter will be distinctly

31. In the reduction of some of the deeper seated parts of the body from a state of enlargement to their natural size, there is a strong proof of a consent or sympathy existing between the superficial and deeper seated absorbent vessels. When, for instance, a swelled testicle is reduced to its natural size by rubbing mercurial ointment upon the surface of the scrotum which covers it, it cannot be supposed that any part of the ointment comes in contact with the absorbent vessels belonging to the substance of the testicle; yet these absorbents are excited to an increased action by the application of the ointment, and the testicle is at length reduced to its natural size. This effect would seem only capable of being explained upon the principle of a consent or sympathy existing between the absorbents of the scrotum and the absorbents of the substance of the testicle, by which, when the former are stimulated, the latter are roused to an increased action.

felt under the skin; but if it should be deeply seated, it will be felt more obscurely, so as to leave the nature of the disease in some doubt. When, however, it has made further progress, it will become perfectly distinct.

When the cartilages of the larynx are converted into bone, the voice has been remarked to become hoarse, or sometimes to be changed into a whisper. This may be easily explained, by the cartilages of the larynx having lost their flexibility, and therefore being rendered incapable of those finer motions which it is reasonable to imagine must have considerable influence upon the voice. In the cases which I have had an opportunity of examining, the ligaments which join the cartilages together were natural in their structure; had they been changed into bone, all the motions of the larynx would have been lost. It would then have been useless as the chief instrument of voice; but what would be the exact effect of such a change upon various sounds transmitted through the trachea and the larynx, it is extremely difficult to determine. In some instances where the cartilages of the larynx have been converted into bone, there has occurred a total inability of swallowing, which destroyed the patients. Upon examination after death, no disease was observable either in the pharynx or the oesophagus. How this should happen it is very difficult to explain, but it has been observed by Dr. Robertson, the Physician of Greenwich Hospital.

When ulcers have taken place in the cavity of the larynx, there is a fixed pain in the situation of this organ, difficulty of breathing and the patient can only speak in a whisper. This state of the larynx is accompanied with more or less of symptomatic fever.

The symptoms which attend catarrh are too generally known to require being mentioned. When there is a sense of soreness in this disease, passing down the middle of the chest, it arises from a considerable inflammation of the inner membrane of the trachea. This inflammation soon goes off, but the increased secretion from the glands of the trachea often remains for a good while afterwards.

The inflammation of the inner membrane of the trachea, which is sometimes to be found in consumptive patients, continues for a much longer time than in catarrh, and may be said to be chronic.

The symptoms of the croup are, symptomatic fever, difficulty of breathing, a wheezing or choaking noise in inspiration, a hoarse voice, and a sort of ringing sound during coughing; portions of a whitish membrane and pus are at the same time occasionally coughed up. It may perhaps be reasonable to suppose that the whitish membrane is formed by some peculiar action of the blood vessels of the inner surface of the larynx and the trachea, which is superadded to inflammation. In common inflammation of the inner surface of the larynx and trachea, there is merely an increased secretion of mucus, or sometimes of pus; but in the croup an adventitious membrane is always formed. This gives some probability to the supposition which we have made; and it may perhaps serve to explain why the croup is so rarely cured by the means which are known to remove common inflammation.

The symptoms which attend a polypus of the trachea are, difficulty of breathing, a dry cough, and a frequent pulse, but without any signs of inflammation. These, however, would not enable physicians to discriminate this disease from several others, if portions of the polypus were not frequently coughed up. The disease is apt to continue for a great length of time.

The symptoms attending spasmodic stricture of the oesophagus characterize sufficiently the nature of the disease. The difficulty of swallowing is not constant, but occasional. It comes on and goes off suddenly, and these changes are frequent. There is no emaciation of the body, and the person generally seems to be in good health.

The stricture of the oesophagus which depends upon the puckering of the inner membrane, is slow in its progress. It may continue for a great many years, and the person seems to be in good health, except for the difficulty of swallowing. The difficulty is constant, which will distinguish it from a mere spasmodic contraction of the muscular fibres of the oesophagus.

The symptoms which belong to a stricture of the oesophagus depending on a scirrhous thickening and ulcer, distinguish it sufficiently from the other two diseases. The difficulty of swallowing is small at first, and gradually becomes worse but is constant. When the disease has made considerable progress, the food is frequently rejected, and along with it occasionally there passes up some pus. The pulse at first is natural, but in the advanced stages of the complaint, is frequent; and towards its termination the body becomes extremely emaciated. The parts in the neighbourhood of the disease are irritated to an increased secretion, which often produces a cough or hawking. Although hardly any nourishment, towards the end of this disease, can be got into the stomach, yet the feeling of hunger is described as not being distressing.

Where there is a fungus or a scrofulous tumour in the oesophagus, the symptoms correspond, I believe, very much with those of the scirrhous stricture of the oesophagus just described.

CHAPTER VI

DISEASED APPEARANCES WITHIN THE CAVITY OF THE ABDOMEN

Ascites

ASCITES, or dropsy of the cavity of the abdomen, is a very frequent disease, and is not confined to any sex or age. I have seen several instances of it in children under ten years old; but it is much more common at the middle, and the more advanced periods of life. It is also more common in the male than the female sex. When water is accumulated in a large quantity in the cavity of the abdomen, the superficial veins of the belly are generally a good deal distended with blood; this probably arises from the pressure of the water upon the deeper seated veins; but it is sometimes hardly observable, even when the accumulation of the water is very considerable. The skin at the navel is also often protruded, yielding easily to pressure, but this is not universally the case. On many occasions the protrusion can hardly be seen, though the water be accumulated in large quantity.

In opening into the cavity of the abdomen, there is to be seen a larger or less quantity of an aqueous fluid, generally of a brownish colour, but its colour varies according to circumstances. When there is a scirrhous liver accompanying the dropsy, the water is commonly of a yellowish or greenish colour. This arises from a mixture of the bile with the water, and under such circumstances there is almost always a jaundiced colour of the skin. I have seen the water in ascites of a chocolate or coffee colour; but this appearance is rare. In the case to which I allude, the water is thicker than that of ascites usually is; but it had the common properties, as far as could be known from the application of heat and of ascids. When none of the viscera of the abdomen are diseased the water in ascites resembles the serum of the blood in its colour, as well as in its other properties.

While water is accumulated in the cavity of the abdomen, the intestinal canal is frequently found to be somewhat in a contracted state; but often too this is not observable. In many cases of ascites the liver is diseased, being hard and tuberculated, as we shall explain particularly when treating of the diseases of the liver. In some cases too, the spleen has been found to be enlarged and hard.

The ascites is not necessarily connected with the accumulation of water any where else in the body; but it frequently happens that it is accompanied with the accumulation of water in the chest, and under the skin, particularly of the lower extremities.

Inflammation of the Peritonaeum

The peritonaeum is not uncommonly inflamed, although it is by no means so liable to this disease as the pleura. There is a cause of inflammation in it peculiar to women, which depends on a certain state of the womb after parturition; but there is also a variety of causes producing it, which are equally applicable to both sexes, so that it is frequently found in men, and also in women who have not been pregnant.

When inflammation has taken place in the peritonaeum, several appearances are observable in opening the body. The peritonaeum is thicker than in its natural state, more pulpy, and less transparent, and it is crowded with a number of very small vessels, containing a florid blood When a portion of the inflamed peritonaeum is separated from the abdominal muscles, there is commonly no appearance whatever of the inflammation having spread into the muscles; but where the peritonaeum covers the intestinal canal, the inflammation is sometimes found to have penetrated not only into the muscular coat of the intestines, but even into the villous membrane. The reason of this difference probably is, that the peritonaeum is less connected with the abdominal muscles than with the intestinal canal, so that the inflammation passes less readily from the peritonaeum to the former than the latter part.

Inflammation of the peritonaeum is sometimes slight and partial; at other times is great and spread over the whole membrane. When it is slight, and affects that part of the peritonaeum which is connected with the intestinal canal, it often forms broad surfaces of inflammation, which run like bands along the course of the intestines, and are bounded by the contact of different portions of the intestines among themselves. In this case the coats of the intestines are not thicker than usual, the inflammation being slight, and confined to the peritonaeum itself. Where the inflammation is great, the intestines are much thicker, and more massy. This evidently arises from the greater accumulation of blood in the small blood vessels, as well as from the extravasation of fluids into the substance of the intestines in consequence of the strong inflammatory action of the vessels. The mesentery and mesocolon are much thicker than in their natural state, and there is also a remarkable change in the omentum. It is frequently as thick as a person's hand, and lies as a circumscribed mass along the greater curvature of the stomach. The principal cause of this change in these parts, is the extravasation of the coagulable lymph into the cellular membrane between the laminae of the peritonaeum which form them.

In many places there is thrown out a layer of a yellowish pulpy matter, gluing different portions of the viscera together. This layer is sometimes thin; at other times is of considerable thickness, and appears to be the coagulable lymph of the blood. There is also a considerable quantity of a brownish fluid in the cavity of the abdomen resembling the serum, which is mixed with small shreds of the coagulable lymph, and sometimes with pus, giving it a turbid appearance. The quantity of the coagulable lymph, and of the fluid, is sometimes large, in proportion to the degree of the inflammation. In some instances, instead of serum a large quantity of pus is found. Air too is sometimes accumulated in the stomach and the intestinal canal, which had been formed in the progress of the disease. At other times this air is wanting. The accumulation of air is most common when the inflammation is slight, and passes in bands along the surface of the intestines.

Adhesions in the Cavity of the Abdomen

When there has been inflammation of the peritonaeum either

generally or partially, sufficient to have thrown out coagulable lymph, and the patient has survived the disease, the coagulable lymph is changed into a fine transparent membrane, which is the membrane of adhesions. The time which is occupied in the change of the coagulable lymph into the membrane of adhesions, is not very long; for I have had several opportunities of tracing the gradual progress of the change from the one into the other, while the inflammation appeared to have been recent. This membrane consists of a cellular substance, similar to the general cellular membrane of the body, and has a moderate share of vascularity. It does not naturally shew many vessels large enough to admit the red globules of the blood; but it shews its vascularity upon slight degrees of inflammation, or when its vessels have been filled with the fine injection. This membrane is capable of elongating gradually by the motion of the viscera upon themselves, so as ultimately to be attended with very little inconvenience. I have very often had an opportunity of observing these adhesions, either joining all the viscera of the abdomen more or less together, or joining some particular viscera to each other.

Scrofulous Masses adhering to the Peritonaeum

I have several times had an opportunity of observing a white soft granulated matter adhering universally behind the peritonaeum. In some places it formed a mass of considerable thickness; in others, it was scattered in single small masses. In one case I recollect that it formed a substance as thick as my hand, between the peritonaeum and the abdominal muscles, while it was scattered in small separate portions in the mesentery and the peritonaeum, covering the intestinal canal. The omentum I have sometimes seen changed into a cake of this substance. The matter itself appears to be scrofulous, for it resembles exactly the structure of a scrofulous absorbent gland before pus is actually formed. I am not at all certain how far this appearance of disease should have been classed along with those of the peritonaeum: it does not take place (at least in the cases which I have seen) in the peritonaeum itself, but behind it, yet at the same time adhering to it. It appears, however, upon the whole to be placed here with more propriety than it could have been any where else.

Cancerous Tumours adhering to the Peritonaeum

I have also seen some small cancerous tumours growing from the peritonaeum. These were extremely hard, of a white colour, and resembled exactly in their structure the cancerous masses which are formed in the stomach. What puts the appearance I allude to beyond doubt, is, that in the same body I found a cancerous tumour of the stomach.

The cancerous tumours of the peritonaeum were not at all connected with this other, but were in that part of the membrane which lines the recti abdominis muscles, nearly opposite to the region of the stomach.

Cartilaginous Excrescences growing from the Peritonaeum

In one case I have seen a great many cartilaginous excrescences growing from the peritonaeum. They were of a small size, viz. most of them not larger than a garden pea, and grew from every part of the membrane. They were a little softer than the cartilages which cover the extremities of the bones, but had the true structure of cartilage.

Steatomatous Tumours adhering to the Peritonaeum

Steatomatous tumours have also been observed adhering to the peritonaeum; but these are of very rare occurrence (32).

Hydatids in the Abdomen

Hydatids have occasionally been found to occupy a portion, or even the whole, of the cavity of the abdomen. In such cases they are connected with the viscera, and chiefly with the liver or the spleen. They may, however, be attached to any viscus or to any part of the peritonaeum. This appearance of disease is uncommon.

---

32. See Soemmerring's German Translation, p. 70.

Air in the Cavity of the Abdomen

Air has been said to be occasionally accumulated in the cavity of the abdomen, while little or none is contained in the intestines (33). This I believe to be a very rare occurrence. Air is not unfrequently accumulated in considerable quantity in the intestinal canal, while there is none at all in the cavity of the abdomen. When a large quantity of air is accumulated in the bowels, they become greatly distended, and their coats proportionably thin. By the bowels lying in close contact with the peritonaeum which lines the muscular parites of the abdomen, there is the same feeling of distension when the hand is pressed against the surface of the belly, and the same quick reaction upon removing the hand, as if the cavity of the belly itself had been filled with air. This has probably given rise to the opinion that the air is often contained in the cavity of the belly. I can believe, however, that air may on some occasions be accumulated in the cavity of the belly, but this is very uncommon. A part of the intestine when very much distended with air may burst, and a portion of the air may escape into the cavity of the belly; or the small arteries of the peritonaeum may secrete air in the same manner as it appears to be formed by the inner membrane of the stomach and the intestine.

SYMPTOMS

The symptoms which belong to ascites are almost too well known to require being mentioned. There is commonly a distinct feeling of fluctuation upon applying one hand to the belly, and striking it with the other; the urine is in small quantity, and of a deep colour; there is thirst, often some feeling of heat, and a pulse more frequent than in health. The breathing is likewise difficult when the water is accumulated in very large quantity.

The symptoms attending inflammation of the peritonaeum are a pain in the abdomen, together with some swelling there, and a great sense of soreness to the touch. The bowels are often costive,

---

33. Vid. Lieutaud, Tom. I. p. 432.

the pulse is frequent and hard, and there are the other circumstances of symptomatic fever strongly marked. When the inflammation is slight, I have known the pain to be very inconsiderable, and the pulse to be little increased in its frequency, so that inflammation of the peritonaeum had not been suspected. Upon examination, however, of the body after death, no other diseased appearance than a slight inflammation of the peritonaeum was discoverable.

There are no symptoms which mark the existence of adhesions in the abdomen; and they seem to be attended with no inconvenience to the functions which are carried on in that cavity.

The symptoms which belong to scrofulous and scirrhous tumours of the peritonaeum are unknown to me.

I know of no symptoms produced by cartilaginous excrescences growing from the peritonaeum. It is probable that they are generally not observable, or not capable of being discriminated.

When hydatids are accumulated in large quantity in the abdomen, it will require some attention to distinguish this disease from ascites. It may be distinguished however in the following manner. In the case of hydatids, the feeling of fluctuation upon striking the belly with the hand will either take place very indistinctly, or not at all: whereas in ascites attended with no extraordinary symptoms, it is always distinct. The swelling in ascites is always uniform, but in an accumulation of hydatids it will be more or less unequal. In hydatids it will be found, upon enquiry into the history of the case, that the swelling first began in some determined place, whereas in ascites there is a gradual swelling of the whole belly.

It will be more difficult to distinguish an accumulation of hydatids from a dropsy of the ovarium than from ascites. The distinction between the two diseases would seem only capable of being determined by an accurate inquiry into the history of the case. In dropsy of the ovarium the swelling is first perceived on the side of the lower part of the belly, and gradually increases upwards, so as to occupy a great part of the cavity of the abdomen. As hydatids most commonly grow from the liver, the swelling in this case will generally be first sensible at the upper part of the belly, and spread downwards. Hydatids, however, may be formed in any part of the abdomen, and therefore were they to begin to be formed at the side of the lower part of the belly, it seems hardly possible to distinguish the one disease from the other.

CHAPTER VII

DISEASED APPEARANCES OF THE STOMACH

Inflammation

It sometimes happens, although not very frequently (unless poisons have been swallowed) that inflammation takes place in the stomach, and spreads over a very considerable portion of its inner membrane, or perhaps the whole of it. It is much more common for inflammation to occupy a smaller portion of the stomach. In such cases the inflammation is generally not very violent. The stomach upon the outside, at the inflamed part, shews a greater number of small vessels than usual, but is commonly not much crowded with them. On opening into the stomach, it is found to be a little thicker at the inflamed part, the inner membrane is very red from the number of small florid vessels, and there are generally spots of extravasated blood. It does not often occur that a common inflammation of the stomach proceeds to form pus, or to terminate in gangrene.

When arsenic has been swallowed (which is the poison most frequently taken) the stomach is affected with a most intense degree of inflammation. Its substance becomes thicker, and there is a very great degree of redness in the inner membrane, arising partly from the very great number of minute vessels, and partly from extravasated blood. Portions of the inner membrane are sometimes destroyed, from the violent action that has taken place in consequence of the immediate application of the poison. I have also seen a thin layer of coagulable lymph thrown out upon a portion of the inner surface of the stomach. Most commonly too, some part of the arsenic is to be seen in the form of a white powder, lying upon different portions of the inner membrane. I have been informed, that in two cases where arsenic had been swallowed, and had destroyed the persons by producing violent inflammation of the stomach, ulcers were found upon examination after death, at the lower end of the rectum. These persons had never complained of any disease in the rectum previously to swallowing the arsenic, and were apparently in good health. This circumstance is very extraordinary, but it is stated from good authority; and it is well worth enquiry, how far the rectum is commonly affected by swallowing arsenic. It is possible that some peculiar sympathy may be established between the lower end of the rectum and the stomach, where violent inflammation has been produced by swallowing this poison, and that the effect of this sympathy may be the formation of an ulcer in that part of the great intestines.

Appearances in the Hydrophobia

On opening the bodies of persons who have died from hydrophobia, the inner membrane of the stomach is frequently found inflamed at the cardia, and its great end. The inner membrane of the pharynx and the oesophagus is also inflamed. The membrane is not thickened by the inflammation, but the inflammation spreads as in erysipelas, shewing in some places a distinct line of boundary. This inflammation I believe is commonly not violent.

Ulcers of the Stomach

Opportunities occasionally offer themselves of observing ulcers of the stomach. These sometimes resemble ulcers in any other part of the body, but frequently they have a peculiar appearance. Many of them are scarcely surrounded with any inflammation, have not irregular eroded edges as ulcers have generally, and are not attended with any particular diseased alteration in the structure of the stomach in the neighbourhood. They appear very much as if, some little time before, a part had been cut out from the stomach with a knife, and the edges had healed, so as to present an uniform smooth boundary round the excavation which had been made. These ulcers sometimes destroy only a portion of the inner coat of the stomach at some one part, but occassionally they destroy a portion of all the coats, forming a hole in the stomach. When a portion of all the coats is destroyed, there is sometimes a thin appearance of the stomach surrounding the hole, which has a smooth surface, and depends on the progress of the ulceration. At other times, the stomach is a little thickened round the hole; and at other times still, it seems to have the common natural structure.

Scirrhous and Cancer of the Stomach

This affection of the stomach is not very uncommon towards an advanced period of life, and I think is more frequently met with in men than in women. This may probably depend upon the greater intemperance in the one sex than in the other.

Scirrhous sometimes extends over almost every part of the stomach, but most commonly it attacks one part. The part which is affected with scirrhous has sometimes no very distinct limit between it and the sound structure of the stomach, but most commonly the limit is very well marked. When scirrhous attacks a portion of the stomach only, it is generally towards the pylorus. The principal reason of this probably is, that there is more of glandular structure in that part of the stomach than in any other; and it would appear that glandular parts of the body are more liable to be affected with scirrhous than other parts.

When the whole stomach, or a portion of it, is scirrhous, it is much thicker than usual, as well as much harder in its texture. When the diseased part is cut into, the original structure of the stomach is frequently marked with sufficient distinctness, but very much altered from the natural appearance. The peritonael covering of the stomach is many times thicker than it ought to be, and has almost a gristly hardness. The muscular part is also very much thickened, and is intersected by numerous membranous septa. These membranous septa are, probably, nothing else than the cellular membrane intervening between the fasciculi of the muscular fibres, thickened from disease. The inner membrane is also extremely thick and hard, and not unfrequently somewhat tuberculated or irregularly elevated towards the cavity of the stomach.

It frequently happens that this thickened mass is ulcerated upon its surface, and then a stomach is said to be cancerous. Sometimes the inner membrane of the stomach throws out a process which terminates in a great many smaller processes, and produces what has been commonly called a fungous appearance.

It also happens that the stomach at some part loses entirely all vestige of its natural structure, and is changed into a very hard mass, of a whitish colour, with some appearance of membrane intersecting it: or it is converted into a gristly substance, like cartilage somewhat softened. The absorbent glands in the neighbourhood are at the same time commonly enlarged, and have a very hard, white structure.

Circumscribed scirrhous Tumours in the Stomach

I have seen several instances of a scirrhous tumour being formed in the stomach about the size of a walnut, while every other part of it was healthy. This tumour has most frequently a small depression near the middle of its surface. While it remains free from irritation, the functions of the stomach are probably very little affected by it; when, however, it is irritated, it must occasion very considerable disorder in the functions of the stomach, and perhaps lay the foundation of a fatal disease.

Pouch formed in the Stomach

A part of the stomach is occasionally formed into a pouch by mechanical means, although very rarely. I have seen one instance of a pouch being so formed, in which five half pence had been lodged. The coats of the stomach were thinner at that part, but were not inflamed or ulcerated. The half pence had remained there for some considerable time, forming a pouch by their pressure, but had not irritated the stomach in such a manner as to produce inflammation or ulceration.

Stricture at the Pylorus

The orifice of the stomach may be almost, or perhaps entirely, shut up by a permanent contraction of its muscular fibres, either at the cardia or the pylorus. This is more likely however, to occur oftenest at the pylorus, because the fibres at this end of the stomach are more circular in their direction, and possess a stronger contractile power. Less contraction too, at the pylorus, will produce an obstruction in the canal, than at the cardia. I have seen one instance of this contraction at the pylorus, which, even there, is a very rare disease. The contraction was so great as hardly to admit a common goose quil to pass from the stomach into the duodenum, and it had prevented a number of plumb stones from passing, which were therefore detained in the stomach.

Stomach much contracted, or much enlarged

The stomach is sometimes found so contracted through the whole of its extent as not to be larger than a portion of the small intestine; and sometimes it is enlarged to much more than its ordinary size. Neither of these appearances are to be considered as arising from disease. They depend entirely on the muscular fibres of the stomach being in a state of contraction or relaxation at the time of death. It happens, I think, more frequently that the stomach is dilated than contracted.

Stomach distended with Air

The stomach is very commonly found, in a dead body, flaccid and almost empty; but not unfrequently it is found more or less distended with air: this air may have been formed after death, but it is often formed during life. When this is the case we may suppose it to be produced by a new chemical arrangement of the contents of the stomach; but it also frequently happens that air is separated from the blood in the blood vessels of the stomach, and poured by the small exhalents into its cavity. This has been more particularly taken notice of by Mr. Hunter, in his Essay upon Digestion (34), and by myself, in a paper which is published in the Medical and Chirurgical Transactions (35).

---

34. See Mr. Hunter's Observations on certain parts of the animal economy, p. 164.
35. See case of emphysema, p. 202.

Part of the Stomach dissolved by the Gastric Juice

In looking upon the coats of the stomach at its great end, a small portion of them there appears frequently to be thinner, more transparent, and feels somewhat more pulpy than is usual; but these appearances are seldom very strongly marked. They arise from the gastric juice resting on that part of the stomach in greater quantity than on any other, and dissolving a small portion of its coats. This is therefore not to be considered as the consequence of a disease, but as a natural effect, depending upon the action of the gastric juice on the coats of the stomach after death. When the gastric juice has been in considerable quantity, and of an active nature, the stomach has been dissolved quite through its substance at the great end, and its contents have been effused into the general cavity of the abdomen. In such cases the neighbouring viscera are also partially dissolved. The instances, however, of so powerful a solution are rare, and have almost only occurred in persons who while in good health had died suddenly from accident. If the powers of the stomach were little impaired by diseases, this appearance of the stomach after death would be very common. As, however, they are very much injured by most diseases, and by many are totally destroyed, this appearance very seldom takes place. The true explanation of these appearances was first given by Mr. Hunter, and published at the request of Sir John Pringle, in the Phylosophical Transactions (36).

Fatty Tumours in the Stomach

Tumours, consisting of a fatty substance, have been sometimes found in the stomach, but they are to be considered as a very rare appearance of disease. Ruysch relates that he has seen a tumour from the stomach of a man which contained hair, together with some dentes molares; and that he has preserved this in his collection (37).

36. See Philosoph. Transact. Vol. 62, p. 447.
37. Vid. Ruysch. Tom. 2. Adversar. Anatomicor. Decad. Tert.

Calculi in the Stomach

Calculi with different appearances have been described as being occasionally found in the stomach. They have never come under my own observation, and are to be reckoned very uncommon (38). Most of these calculi have been found upon examination to be biliary, and had been conveyed from the duodenum into the stomach by an antiperistaltic motion of this part of the small intestines.

Morbid Papillae observed in the Stomach

Papillae and pustules, somewhat resembling the small-pox, have also been described as being formed on the inner membrane of the stomach, but these are exceedingly rare (39).

Small-pox Pustules said to be in the Stomach

Even true small-pox pustules have been said to be found in the stomach of persons who died from this disease (40). In later dissections, however, this appearance has not been observed, and I am disposed to believe, where it has been thought to exist, that some mistake has been made.

SYMPTOMS

In inflammation of the stomach, the following symptoms are observed to take place: viz. pain in the epigastric region, which is increased when anything has been swallowed, vomiting, often hickup, symptomatic fever with a small, frequent, and hard pulse, and a feeling of great debility.

The symptoms which are produced by swallowing arsenic, are the same with those which take place in a very violent inflammation of the stomach; for arsenic acts upon that organ in no other way than by exciting in it a very high degree of inflammation.

---

38. Vid. Lieutaud, Tom. I. p. 17.
39. Vid. Lieutaud, Tom. I. p. 23.
40. Vid. Lieutaud, Tom. I. p. 371.

Hydrophobia is sufficiently characterized by the horror which the patient expresses at the sight of any fluid that is offered to him, by the great difficulty experienced in swallowing, and by the strong alienation of mind which accompanies this dreadful disease.

I have reason to believe that ulcers of the stomach are often slow in their progress. They are attended with pain, or an uneasy feeling in the stomach, and what is swallowed is frequently rejected by vomiting.

This state continues for a considerable length of time, and is very little relieved by medicine; which may serve as some ground of distinction between the complaint and a temporary deranged action of the stomach.

Cancer of the stomach is attended with a sense of pain in that organ, which varies a good deal in its degree in different individuals. What is swallowed is commonly rejected by vomiting, and there is frequently thrown up a dark coloured fluid, which has sometimes been compared to coffee grounds. The patient becomes at length emaciated, and the countenance sallow; the pulse at the beginning of this dreadful complaint is natural, but towards the close of it is frequent, and is accompanied with the usual symptoms of hectic fever. Where the person is much emaciated, and the cancerous swelling is situated near the pylorus or along a part of the great curvature of the stomach, it may be felt, if its bulk be considerable, by a careful examination with the hand in the living body.

The accumulation of air in the stomach, is accompanied with an unpleasant feeling of distention there, and a swelling may be felt externally in the epigastric region; wind passes up by the oesophagus, and there are occasional pains in the stomach produced by a spasmodic contraction of some part of its muscular coat.

CHAPTER VIII

DISEASED APPEARANCES IN THE INTESTINES

Inflammation

THE intestinal canal is subject to inflammation from a variety of causes, and therefore we have frequent opportunities of observing its effects after death. When a portion of intestine is inflamed, there is spread upon its outer surface a number of small vessels, many of which contain florid blood. When the intestine is cut into, so as to exhibit its inner membrane, this appears highly vascular from the small vessels of the villi being loaded with blood, and there are frequently to be seen in it a few spots of blood extravasated. In inflammation of the intestines, the peritonaeum is often very little, or not at all affected. When, however, the inflammation is very great, the peritonaeum is also inflamed, and covered with a layer of coagulable lymph. I have likewise seen, in violent inflammation, scattered portions of coagulable lymph thrown out upon the surface of the villous membrane; this however is very uncommon. The intestine is at the same time much more thick and massy than in a healthy state, and its colour is sometimes very dark from a large quantity of black extravasated blood. This state of the intestine has often been mistaken for mortification.

It very commonly happens that inflammation of the intestines advances to suppuration and ulceration. This takes place where the inflammation is confined principally to the inner membrane of the intestines. The ulcer is formed upon the inner surface; and I do not recollect to have seen one instance where the ulcer had begun upon the outer surface of the intestines and had spread inwards. Ulceration, however, does not appear to be so common in the small as in the great intestines. When it takes place either in the one or the other intestine, it is attended with considerable variety in its appearance: the edges of the ulcer have sometimes considerable thickness; and sometimes they are not thicker than the healthy structure of the intestine; the edges and general cavity of an ulcer are sometimes ragged and at other times they are smooth, as if a portion had been cut out from the intestine with a knife. Sometimes through a considerable length of the intestine (especially if it be the great one) the inner membrane hangs in tattered shreds, occasioned by the great ravage of the ulceration. I have also seen a considerable portion of the intestine completely stripped of its inner membrane, from the extent of this process, and its muscular coat appeared as distinct as if the inner membrane had been very carefully dissected off. In the follicular glands, which are gathered together in little oval groups, I think ulceration occurs more frequently than in the other parts of the intestine.

When ulceration advances very actively, it sometimes eats through the coats of the intestine entirely. When this is the case, a portion of the contents of the intestine occasionally passes into the general cavity of the abdomen, producing inflammation there. This, however, does not very often happen; most commonly that portion of the gut where the ulcer is situated, adheres by inflammation to some other portion, or to a neighbouring viscus, and a communication is formed between the one and the other. I have seen communications formed in this manner between the rectum and the bladder in a male, and between the rectum and the vagina in a female. I have even seen a communication formed between the kidney and a portion of the intestine from this cause, by which the pus produced in the kidney was evacuated through the intestine. Such communications are the means of preserving life (although in a very uncomfortable state,) for a much longer time than it could be, were the matter to pass into the general cavity of the belly. It would there produce peritonael inflammation, which would soon destroy. The inner membrane of the intestines is more disposed to become ulcerated, than the inner membrane of any other canal which has an external opening. Thus ulcers are very rare in the inner membrane of the trachea or the urethra, but very common in the inner membrane both of the great and the small intestines. It is difficult to assign a satisfactory reason for this difference. It probably, however, depends upon the different structures and functions of these parts. There is a good deal of resemblance between the structure of the inner membrane of the trachea and the urethra. The secretion of the one, likewise, is not very different from that of the other. The inner membrane of the intestines has a structure and secretion peculiar to itself. It is probable that upon these circumstances depends its greater dispostion to ulcerate; but it is very difficult to explain how this should be the case.

Inflammation of the intestines sometimes, although rarely, advances to mortification. When this is the case, the mortified part is of a dark livid colour, and has lost its tenacity; it is in this state very easily torn through, or the fingers will pass through it as through a rotten pear. The want of the natural tenacity, when attended with the change of colour which we have mentioned, is the only sure criterion of a part being mortified, in examinations after death. A portion of intestine may be of a very dark colour, and yet may not be mortified. This darkness of colour may be occasioned by a large quantity of extravasated blood thrown out during a high degree of inflammation, where the principle of life is maintained in full vigour. Thus we see blood, effused into the cellular membrane under the skin, producing a very dark appearance, yet the parts are quite alive. It has often happened, too, that a very dark portion of intestine has been returned in the operation of the bubonocele, and yet the parts have recovered their natural functions. This could never have happened if the black portion of the intestine had really been mortified. Under such circumstances, the mortified part would have separated from the living, and the function of the gut must have been destroyed. When a portion of gut has been for some time mortified, a considerable quantity of air is formed, which is accumulated in its cavity. This is a part of the natural process which takes place in all dead animal substances. I have known an instance where a large portion of the great intestine (viz. above a yard of it,) had lost its living principle, and was expelled through the anus. The person lived about three weeks afterwards (41).

---

41. See Medical and Chirurgical transactions, Vol. 2. p. 144.

Intus-Susceptio

This is not a very uncommon disease, and is frequently fatal. It consists in a portion of gut passing for some length within another portion, and dragging along with it a part of the mesentery. The portion of gut which is received into the other, is in a contracted state, and is sometimes of considerable length. It usually happens that an upper portion of intestine falls into a lower; but the contrary likewise occurs, although rarely. Intus-susceptio may take place in any part of the intestinal canal, but it happens most frequently in the small intestines, and where the ileum terminates in the colon. In this last situation, it appears to me to happen more frequently than any where else. This, perhaps, depends on the great difference in size between these two portions of intestine. In opening bodies, particularly of infants, an intus-susceptio is not unfrequently found, which had been attended with no mischief: the parts appear perfectly free from inflammation, and they would probably have been easily disentangled from each other by their natural peristaltic motion. At other times, however, so large a portion of the gut passes within another portion of it that it cannot be disentangled, which may produce violent inflammation, and the passage of the intestines is obstructed, without any possibility of its being set free. This is the fatal state of the disease.

Ruptures

A portion of the viscera of the abdomen frequently passes out of that cavity, being lodged in a bag of elongated peritonaeum; and this disease is called a rupture. It happens most commonly from some sudden and violent concussion of the body, where the weaker parts of the parietes of the abdomen give way. I once thought, and it is I believe the general opinion, that ruptures occur more frequently in fat than in lean people; but from some conversation which I have had with persons, whose line of life leads them to give particular attention to this disease, I am disposed to think that this opinion is ill founded. Ruptures are found to be as frequent in persons who are not corpulent, as in those who are (42).

There is hardly any viscus which has not at some time or other, been found in the sack of a rupture, but most frequently it is either a portion of the omentum, or of the intestines, or of both. The bag formed by the peritonaeum may be thrust out almost at any part of the belly; but this happens most frequently at the ring of the external oblique muscle, under Paupart's ligament, and at the navel: it also sometimes takes place at other parts of the abdomen. There is another situation where a rupture has been known to happen, although very rarely, viz. through an opening in the diaphragm into the thorax. The opinion which would most obviously be formed about this is, that a portion of the diaphragm had burst and a part of the intestines had protruded into the opening made in the diaphragm. I am persuaded, however, that this opinion will almost always be ill founded. It happens sometimes, but very seldom, that children are born with a hole in the diaphragm, which is a malformation or monstrosity in this part of the body. When the hole is large, a considerable portion of the abdominal viscera passes into the thorax, and so impedes the functions of the heart and lungs, that children under these circumstances perish immediately after birth. When the hole in the diaphragm is small, it lays the foundation of the hernia or rupture which we have just described, and which may be called, by way of distinction, the diaphragmatic hernia (43).

It is well known that the most usual situation of a rupture in the male, is at the ring of the external oblique muscle; and this arises probably from the larger size of that opening in the male than in the female. The most usual situation of a rupture in the female is known also to be either under Paupart's ligament, or at the navel. The reason of the frequency of the first situation, is the particular shape of the pelvis in the female, by which there is a larger empty space under Paupart's ligament, than in the male, so that the viscera in that part are less firmly supported. The reason

42. The umbilical rupture should be considered as an exception to this remark, for it is much more common in fat people than those of a spare habit.

43. A case of this kind has occurred to Dr. Clarke, and has been published by him in the 2nd volume of the Medical and Chirurgical Transactions, p. 118. He has been so obliging as to give me the preparation which illustrates this hernia.

why the second situation of a rupture occurs often in a female, is, probably, frequent child-bearing. During pregnancy, at its advanced period, the navel opens, or gives way, and where pregnancies have been frequent, it probably never recovers its original strength.

The omentum is more commonly found in the sack of a rupture than any of the viscera. This perhaps arises from its being a loose mass, not tied down to any particular situation, and therefore it readily passes into any cavity which communicates with the abdomen. When it has once fallen down, it has no means of pulling itself out, like a portion of intestine, which is another reason why it is so often found in a rupture. When it has remained long in a sack, it forms a pretty compact mass, sometimes having no connection with, but at other times adhering to the inner surface of the sack. There is frequently no inflammation produced in the omentum while in this situation, but occasionally violent inflammation takes place, which may even advance to mortification.

A portion of gut is very often lodged in the sack of a rupture, either by itself, or along with a portion of the omentum. The portion of gut is sometimes very small, but sometimes it is very considerable. Very often the functions of the intestines go on properly in this situation, but occasionally violent inflammation is produced, interrupting their function, and often terminating fatally. This inflammation is produced by the gut being strongly pressed at the narrowest part of the sack, viz. at that part where the sack immediately passes out of the cavity of the abdomen. This inflammation exhibits the different appearances, upon dissection, which we have so often related. The gut too, is frequently found mortified: this is shewn by its dark colour, by its want of proper tenacity, and by the air which is formed within it. When the inflammation of the gut in a sack has not been very violent, and has terminated by resolution, it frequently leaves adhesions behind it, connecting the gut with the inner surface of the sack. It is perhaps possible too, that adhesions may be formed by long close contact, without inflammation.

When the sack of a rupture has not been of long standing, it consists of a thin, firm, white, opaque membrane; this is a protruded part of the peritonaeum, somewhat thickened by pressure (44). When the sack has been of long standing, it is often very thick, and evidently consists of a number of layers. The sack upon the inside has a very smooth surface, and the membrane which forms this surface, can be readily traced into the peritonaeum, lining the cavity of the abdomen; the outer surface of the sack is more rough and coarse in its texture. The sack, where it passes out of the cavity of the abdomen, has frequently a narrow neck, or aperture, and is distended below into a bag of considerable size. At other times, the communication between the sack and the cavity of the abdomen is by a larger opening.

Hernia Congenita

In bubonocele the sack is usually quite distinct from the sack of the tunica vaginalis testis. Sometimes, however, there is no separation between them, and the contents of the rupture are immediately in contact with the body of the testicle: this kind of rupture is called hernia congenita. It was formerly supposed to arise from a portion of the sack of the rupture and of the tunica vaginalis giving way, so that the contents of the rupture fell into the cavity of the tunica vaginalis testis, and came in contact with the testicle. Upon a little reflection, it might have been perceived that this could hardly take place; though the true account of this appearance was not known till it was explained by Dr. Hunter. Baron Haller discovered, that till about the eighth month the testicles do not descend into the scrotum, but are situated in the cavity of the abdomen under the kidneys. When they descend into the scrotum, the peritonaeum that covers them is necessarily drawn down along with them through the ring of the external oblique muscle; it then forms a bag, the upper extremity of which communicates with the cavity of the abdomen. Baron Haller had also observed, that in infants a portion of intestine sometimes falls down into this bag after the testicle, or along with it, producing what he called the hernia congenita. The communication between

44. In some cases of umbilical hernia, Dr. Marshall has observed no distinct appearance of peritonaeal sack. This must have arisen from the peritonaeum having burst, in consequence of distention, and its ruptured edges being lost by adhesion in the neighbouring parts.

the bag and the abdomen is commonly closed, sometimes a little before, and sometimes soon after birth. It appears, however, that if it be prevented from closing at the usual time, it does not close afterwards but remains open through life. Hence, if any portion of an intestine, or of the omentum, falls into the elongated sack of the peritonaeum, it must be in contact with the testicle. When Dr. Hunter became acquainted with the observations of Baron Haller upon the descent of the testicles, he saw at once that the species of rupture sometimes to be met with in adults, where a portion of intestine or omentum is in contact with the testicle, might be easily explained. His explanation corresponded with that which we have just given, and has been universally adopted by anatomists and surgeons.

Schirrhus and Cancer of the Intestines

Schirrhus is a disease which takes place much more commonly in the great than in the small intestines, but the latter are occasionally affected by it. I have seen a schirrhus tumour, and a cancerous ulcer in the duodenum. In the great intestine, at an advanced period of life, schirrhus is not uncommon: every portion of this intestine is not equally liable to be affected by it, but it is to be found much more frequently at the sigmoid flexure of the colon, or in the rectum, than any where else, which perhaps may depend on the following circumstances. There is certainly more of glandular structure in the inner membrane of the great intestines towards its lower extremity, than in any other part of it, and this sort of structure has a greater tendency to be affected with schirrhus, than the ordinary structures of the body: the gut, too, is narrower at the sigmoid flexure than at any other part, and therefore will be more liable to be injured by the passage of hard bodies; these by their irritation, may excite the disease of schirrhus in a part which was pre-disposed to it.

The schirrhus sometimes extends over a considerable length of the gut, viz. several inches; but generally it is more circumscribed. It exhibits the same appearances of structure which were described when speaking of schirrhus of the stomach. The peritonaeal, muscular, and internal coats are much thicker and harder than in a natural state. The muscular too is subdivided by membraneous septa, and the internal coat is sometimes formed into hard irregular folds. It often happens that the surface of the inner membrane is ulcerated, producing cancer. Every vestige of the natural structure is occasionally lost, and the gut appears changed into a gristly substance. When schirrhus affects the gut, the passage at that part is always narrowed, and sometimes so much so as to be almost entirely obstructed. The obliteration, or stricture, would sometimes appear to be greater than in proportion to the thickness of the sides of the diseased gut: this, most probably, depends upon the contraction of the muscular fibres of the gut, which, although diseased, have not altogether lost their natural action. Where the passage is very much obstructed, the gut is much enlarged immediately above the obstruction, from the accumulation of the contents in that part of the intestine. While this disease is going on in a portion of the intestine, adhesions are formed between it and the neighbouring viscera, and the ulceration sometimes spreads from the one to the other.

The diseased Change of the Intestines in Dysentery

The inner membrane of the great intestines I have seen a good deal thickened, and formed into small irregular tubercles, some of which were of a white, and others of a yellowish colour; the peritonaeal and muscular coats were also thicker and harder than in a natural state. In some places too the inner membrane appeared abraded, and the tubercles were sometimes fissured upon the surface, so as to resemble little common warts. This is not a frequent appearance of disease, but it is generally been found to take place in very severe dysenteries, such as those which occasionally arise in camps. In the common cases of dysentery, which takes place during the autumnal season in this country, the morbid appearance just described is not found; at least no instance of it has fallen under my observation. When such cases prove fatal, a number of ulcers are discovered, by examination after death, in the inner membrane of the great and sometimes of the small intestines.

Thickened Folds of the Inner Membrane of the Great Intestines

I have also seen the internal membrane of the great intestines formed into broad thick folds, in which a considerable quantity of blood was accumulated; these folds were perfectly independent of the state of the contraction in the muscular coat, and were very different in their appearance from the irregular puckering which is often seen in the inner membrane of the great intestines. When these folds were examined, they were found to consist of an accumulation of cellular membrane, with the inner coat of the gut reflected over it.

Upon the inner surface of the great intestine, about two inches above the anus, little processes sometimes grow from the internal membrane; they generally surround the gut at short distances from each other, so as to form a sort of circle.

Piles

Piles, and fistulae in ano, are diseases which are extremely common, but which hardly ever become an object of examination after death; they have therefore not been so commonly introduced into accounts of morbid appearances, as others which much more rarely occur. Piles are soft tumours commonly situated round the verge of the anus, sometimes of a regularly bulbous, and sometimes of an irregular form. They are covered with a very tender skin, which partly consists of the fine skin immediately round the anus on the outside, and partly of the inner membrane of the gut. The tumours are generally entire, but they have occasionally small openings through which a considerable quantity of blood is sometimes poured; they consist commonly of the veins round the verge of the anus, much enlarged from the accumulation of blood. These veins are branches of the internal iliac vein, but they communicate largely with the lower branches of the mesaraica minor.

The same sort of tumours are also frequently found within the cavity of the rectum, forming what have been called the internal piles; and these are occasioned by the enlargement of some of the branches of the mesaraica minor. Piles are a much more frequent disease in persons who are advanced in life, than in those who are young. They arise from repeated, and long continued impediments to the return of the blood from the lower part of the rectum, and there has been much more opportunity for these impediments to act in old, than in young persons. They are also more common in women than in men. This may arise from several causes: the uterus during pregnancy must occasion a great impediment to the return of the blood from the rectum: this is so much the case, that women who have been frequently pregnant seldom escape piles. Women too are more apt to allow of an accumulation of the proper contents of the rectum, than men, which will produce some impediment to the return of the blood from this part.

Fistulae in Ano

Fistulae in ano are narrow canals at the lower end of the rectum, and are distinguished by the following circumstances: they have callous edges, a smooth internal surface, and possess the power of secreting pus (45). A disease of this sort may consist of one canal, opening by a very small aperture externally, at the side of the anus; or this canal may be divided into several branches. The canal, besides opening externally, has very commonly a small opening into the gut itself; and sometimes there is a small opening into the gut, without there being any externally on the side of the anus. It is much more common, however, to find only an external opening of the canal; or, to find both an external opening, and another into the gut.

The Rectum terminating in a Cul-de-sac

It is a species of monstrous formation, not very uncommon, that the rectum does not terminate in the anus, but in a cul-de-sac, without reaching the external surface. Sometimes the extremity of the gut lies near the external surface, but more commonly it is at some distance from it. In these cases there is usually the

45. Mr. Hunter has observed, in his Lectures on Surgery, that fistulae have a smooth internal surface, like a secreting surface, as, for instance, the urethra.

appearance of an anus, but the opening is more contracted than in the natural structure. It seldom happens that this malformation can be effectually remedied by a chirurgical operation. The opening which is made into the extremity of the gut has generally such a disposition to close, that the benefit which might naturally be expected from an operation is frustrated. A few cases however have occurred in which the operation has been successful.

The Rectum terminating in the Bladder

I have also seen the rectum terminate in the bladder from an original error in the formation, so that there was no other external opening to the rectum than by the urethra: this was in a child at birth: the malformation was of such a kind, as neither to admit of a remedy by art, nor to allow of life being continued.

The rectum has also been known to terminate in the vagina, from a defect in the original formation; but this is very uncommon.

Worms

Worms are formed in the intestines of man, as well as of many other classes of animals; but not so frequently in the former as in the latter. In most quadrupeds and fishes it is extremely common to find a number of worms upon opening their intestines.

The worms which are found in the human subject, may be reduced to three general classes, viz. the lumbricus teres; taenia; and ascaris.

Lumbricus Teres

The lumbricus teres, or round worm, is much more commonly found in the intestines of children, than in those of persons full grown, or advanced in life: it is very usually met with in the first, but rarely in the two last. The lumbricus teres is known to differ from the common earth worm, but practitioners in this country have made little inquiry into the circumstances upon which this difference depends. The two species of worms, if attentively examined, will be found to differ a good deal from each other in their external appearance. The lumbricus teres is more pointed at both extremities, than the common earth worm. The mouth of the lumbricus teres consists of three rounded projections, with an intermediate cavity; the mouth of the earth worm consists of a small longitudinal fissure, situated on the under surface of a small rounded head. Upon the under surface too of this worm there is a large semilunar fold of skin, into which the head retreats, or out of which it is elongated, which is entirely wanting in the lumbricus teres. The anus of the lumbricus teres opens upon the under surface of the worm, a little way from its posterior extremity, by a transverse curved fissure; the anus of the earth worm opens by an oval aperture at the very extremity of the worm. The outer covering or skin in the lumbricus teres is less fleshy, and strongly marked by transverse rugae, than in the earth worm. In the latter there is often to be seen a broad yellowish band, surrounding the body of the worm; but in the lumbricus teres, this is entirely wanting. On each side of the lumbricus teres there is a longitudinal line very well marked; in the earth worm there are three longitudinal lines upon the upper half of its surface, but these are so faintly marked, as to be hardly observable. The lumbricus teres has nothing corresponding to feet, whereas the earth worm has on its under surface, but more strongly marked towards its posterior extremity, a quadruple row of processes on each side, very sensible both to the eye, and the finger, which manifestly serve the purposes of feet in the locomotion of the animal.

The internal structure of these two species of worms is also extremely different. In the lumbricus teres, there is an intestinal canal, nearly uniform and smooth in its appearance, which passes from one extremity of the worm to the other. Near the head of this worm, the canal is narrower than it is any where else, and somewhat distinct in its limits: this may be considered as the oesophagus. In the earth worm there is a large and complex stomach, consisting of two cavities; and the intestinal canal in the latter is likewise larger, and more formed into sacculi, than the former. The parts subservient to generation in these two species of worms differ very much from each other; in the lumbricus teres there is a distinction of sex, the parts of generation being different in the male and in the female; in the common earth worm the organs of generation are the same in each individual, as this worm is hermaphrodite. The appearance too of the organs of generation, is extremely different at first sight in the one species of animal, and the other. There is an oval mass situated at the anterior extremity of the earth worm, resembling a good deal the medullary matter of the brain; in the lumbricus teres this substance is wanting (46). These are the principal differences between the one species of animal and the other, which are obvious upon a very moderate attention to each. Many other differences would, doubtless, be found by a person who might choose to prosecute their anatomy minutely.

Taenia

The taenia which is most commonly found in the human intestines, is of two kinds, viz. the taenia solium, and the taenia lata.

Taenia Solium

This taenia is frequently bred in the intestines of the inhabitants of Germany, and occasionally, but rarely, in those of the inhabitants of Great Britain. It consists of a great many distinct portions, which are connected together so as to put on a jointed appearance; these joints are commonly of a very white colour, but are occasionally brownish, which depends on a fluid of this colour that is found in their vessels. The worm is usually very long, extending often many yards, and seldom passes entire from the bowels. This circumstance has prevented the extremities of the taenia from being so often seen.

The head of this taenia is somewhat of a square form, with a narrowed projection forwards; in the middle of this projecting part, there is a distinct circular aperture, around the edge of which grow curved sharp processes. Near the angles of the square edge of the head, are situated four round projecting apertures, at equal

46. What this substance is I do not know, and I have only mentioned its resemblance to the medullary matter of the brain, in order to give a clearer description of it.

distances from each other: this head is placed upon a narrow jointed portion of the worm, of considerable length, and which gradually spreads itself into the broader joints, of which the body of the worm is composed.

The body of the taenia consists of thin, flat, pretty long joints, on one edge of which there is a projection, with a very obvious aperture. In the same worm some of these joints appear considerably longer than others, which probably depends on one joint being contracted, while another is relaxed. The apertures which we have just mentioned are generally placed on the opposite edges of the contiguous joints; but this is not uniformly the case; they are sometimes placed on the same edges of two, or even several contiguous joints. When these joints are examined attentively, there are frequently seen, in each of them, vessels filled with a brownish fluid, and disposed in an arborescent form. Around the edges of each joint, there is also a distinct serpentine canal (47). The last joint of a taenia resembles very much a common joint rounded off at its extremity, and without any aperture.

Taenia Lata

The taenia lata is bred very commonly in the intestines of the inhabitants of Switzerland, but very rarely in those of the inhabitants of Great Britain. The joints of which it is composed are short and broad, and the aperture is not upon the edge of each joint, as in the solium, but in the middle of its flattened surface. Round these apertures are short, radiated vessels. The head is of an oval shape, and so small that its minute structure is not visible by the naked eye. Its tail terminates in two narrow processes, one of which is longer than the other.

Other taenia have occasionally been found in the human intestines, but they occur very rarely, and have not fallen under my own observation.

---

47. This, as well as the vessels disposed in an arborescent form, is very distinctly seen injected in some preparations which have been made, and given to me by an ingenious surgeon, Mr. Carlisle.

Ascaris

The ascaris is a very small worm, which is often found at the lower end of the rectum in children, and even more frequently in adults than is commonly imagined. It is white in its colour, and about half an inch in length; at the extremity where its head is placed, it is a little narrowed, and at the other extremity it terminates in a long, very fine, transparent process. These worms are more or less surrounded with mucus, which is secreted in increased quantity by the glands in the inner membrane of the rectum, from the irritation occasioned by the worms.

Trichuris

This worm has been occasionally found in the great intestines of man, and more especially the coecum. It resembles a good deal the ascaris, but is considerably larger, and has a very long transparent tail. To their heads is attached a process or horn, which they can protrude or retract.

There is nothing in the economy of animals more obscure than the origin of intestinal worms; were they found to live out of the bodies of living animals, one might readily suppose that their ovula were taken into the body along with the food and drink, and there gradually evolved into animals. This, however, is not the case; they do not seem capable of living for any length of time in any situation, except within a living animal body, which appears to be the proper place for their growth and residence. We might therefore be led to another supposition, viz. that intestinal worms are really formed from the matter contained in the intestines, which previously had no regular organization; but this idea is widely different from all analogy in the production of animals, where there has been any satisfactory opportunity of examining this production. The origin, therefore, of such animals is a subject of much obscurity, and probably will not have soon any satisfactory light thrown upon it.

Air accumulated in the Intestines

It is not unusual to find air accumulated in the intestinal canal, in greater or less quantity; this air is sometimes, but not constantly, accompanied with a slight inflammation of the peritonaeum. In such cases, the blood vessels, creeping upon the intestines, are sometimes filled with air, but frequently they are without it. Air is often let loose into the intestines after death by putrefaction: but that which we wish particularly to consider here, has been formed during life.

There are only two ways in which we can well conceive air to be formed in the intestines: the one is, some new arrangement in the contents of the intestines, by which air is extricated: the other is, the formation of air in the blood vessels of the intestines by a process similar to secretion, and which air is afterwards poured out by the extremities of the exhalent arteries into the cavity of the intestines. That the blood vessels of an animal body have this power there can be no doubt; and I own I am inclined to think that this is a mode not unfrequent by which air is accumulated in the intestines. This air probably differs somewhat at different times; in several trials which I have made, it never shewed signs of containing any proportion of inflammable air, but always a very sensible proportion of fixed air. It requires, however, to be examined by some person well acquainted with chemical experiments, in order that its ingredients may be exactly ascertained.

Bony Matter formed in the Intestines

These are the most common appearances of diseased, or preternatural structure in the intestines; but I have likewise had an opportunity of observing others, which are of rarer occurrence. In one or two instances I have seen a sort of bony matter thrown out upon the surface of the inner membrane of the gut: I have even seen an adhesion between two portions of intestine, converted into bone. It would appear, that almost every part of the body is occasionally subject to this process. It may not improperly be considered, as a natural process misplaced. An adhesion being once formed, has the same power (as far as we know) of running into different processes, as the cellular membrane, which makes a part of the original structure. It may therefore form bone, as readily as cellular membrane, or some other membranes of the body, which have a resemblance to the membrane of adhesions, as the pleura and the peritonaeum.

Projecting Ring formed in the Cavity of Jejunum

I have seen one of the valvulae conniventes much larger than usual, and passing round on the inside of the jejunum, like a broad ring. The canal of the gut was necessarily much narrowed at this ring; but no mischief had arisen from it. This malformation, however, might have laid the foundation of fatal mischief. Some substance, too large to pass, might have rested on the ring, and produced their inflammation, ulceration, and ultimately death.

Calculous Matter in the Intestines

Calculous matter has sometimes been known to be accumulated in some part of the cavity of the intestinal canal, especially in the great intestine; but this has not come under my own observation, and, at least in the human subject, is a very rare occurrence (48).

Small-pox Pustules said to be in the Intestines

Small-pox pustules have been said to be sometimes found in the intestines of persons who had died from this disease (49). How far this may have occasionally taken place, I will not pretend to say, but late dissections, upon the best authority, have not confirmed this fact.

Diseased Appearances of the Mesentery—Mesentery inflamed

The mesentery is often found in a state of inflammation; although I believe this hardly ever takes place, unless when the peritonaeum generally is inflamed. When the mesentery is inflamed, it becomes much thicker, and more massy, than in its natural state; the large blood vessels which pass between its laminae and the absorbent glands, are also very much obscured.

48. Vid. Lieutaud, Tom. I. p. 77, 78.
49. Vid. Lieutaud, Tom. I. p. 371.

These different appearances depend upon the quantity of the coagulable lymph which is thrown out, during the inflammatory action. The peritonaeum which forms the laminae of the mesentery is crowded with small blood vessels, and is covered more or less with a layer of the coagulable lymph. A small quantity of pus is sometimes found on the surface of the inflamed mesentery, and even abscesses have been observed between its laminae, but this last appearance is very rare.

It very seldom happens, that the mesentery is found gangrenous, unless different portions of the intestinal canal be found in the same state. When the intestines are mortified, portions of the mesentery are sometimes found in the same condition. The appearances exhibited in mortification are the same when it affects the mesentery, as in any other part, and they have been already described.

Mesenteric Glands scrofulous

The absorbent glands of the mesentery, are frequently found to be scrofulous, and this is more apt to take place in children, than in persons of a more advanced age. When affected with this disease, the glands exhibit different appearances, according to its progress: they are enlarged in their size, and are somewhat softer to the touch, than in a natural state. When cut into, they sometimes shew very much the natural structure; but more frequently they are changed, in part, into a white, soft, curdly matter; and this is not uncommonly mixed with pus.

Mesenteric Glands cancerous

When a portion of the intestinal canal becomes cancerous, some of the absorbent glands in the mesentery generally become affected with the same disease: this is in consequence of the matter of cancer being conveyed to those glands by absorbent vessels. The glands become enlarged in size, and are changed into hard masses exhibiting a schirrhus, or a cancerous structure.

Mesenteric Glands earthy or bony

The absorbent glands of the mesentery are sometimes filled

with an earthy, or bony matter; but this is to be considered as a rare occurrence (50). The absorbent glands at the root of the lungs are more liable to be affected with this disease.

Hydatids have also been occasionally found adhering to the mesentery.

Tumours, likewise, consisting of a fatty matter, have been seen attached to the mesentery; but these I believe to be very uncommon.

SYMPTOMS

Inflammation of the intestines is characterized by the following symptoms, viz. an acute pain in the abdomen, vomiting, obstinate costiveness, symptomatic fever, with a frequent small and hard pulse. The pulse, however, is sometimes less affected than might have been supposed, from the violence of the inflammation.

The symptoms attending intus-susceptio are similar to those which belong to inflammation of the intestines, and indeed this disease is not unfrequently accompanied with inflammation. It is however more likely to prove fatal than simple inflammation of the bowels, as it does not admit of any substantial benefit from medicine.

When there is a rupture without any strangulation of the intestine, the following symptoms take place, viz. a pale swelling at the part affected, a slight pain occasionally felt in the swelling itself, and spread somewhat over the region of the belly, the swelling pushed out by coughing, a disappearance of the swelling upon pressure, or upon the person continuing for a considerable length of time in a horizontal posture. When a rupture is large and of long standing, it will often be incapable of being reduced by pressure, even when there is no strangulation.

When strangulation takes place, the same symptoms arise which belong to inflammation of the bowels, for the strangulation produces inflammation. These consist of a pain in the swelling, which is diffused over the abdomen, sickness, vomiting, obstinate costiveness, heat, commonly a frequent, small, and hard pulse: and

50. Vid. Med. Transactions, Vol. I. p. 361.

towards the fatal conclusion of the disease there is hickup, with a foetid yellow matter thrown out by the mouth. The sickness I have heard described, as being infinitely more distressing than the ordinary sickness of a deranged stomach; the pulse is sometimes, in such a case, not increased in frequency beyond the standard of health; and yet the inflammation of the bowel has been discovered afterwards by the operation to be very great. This is an important practical observation, because it shews that the degree of inflammation is not to be judged of from the pulse, and teaches that the operation should not be delayed, after the proper efforts for reducing the rupture have failed, because the pulse may happen to be little or not at all accelerated.

When the great intestine is attacked with schirrhus, the disease has commonly made some progress, before it is much attended to by the patient. At first there is but little pain in the part affected, and the patient observes that he is costive, or that the stools pass with some difficulty. When the disease is more advanced a considerable pain is felt, more especially in passing a stool, and there are occasional sympathetic pains about the os sacrum and hips. When the stools are examined, they are commonly found to be narrow, to be more or less flattened, and they are sometimes besmeared with mucus, pus, and blood. The pulse at the beginning of this disease is natural, but towards its close becomes accelerated. In advanced stages of the disease, the countenance is sallow, the strength is much impaired, the body is much emaciated, and the constitution at length altogether sinks.

In dysentery, griping pains are felt in the abdomen, which often arise to a considerable degree of severity. The bowels are irritated to frequent evacuation, and generally discharge mucus tinged with blood, but sometimes white lumps, membranous films, pus, and at intervals scybala. Tenesmus accompanies the evacuation of the bowels; and there is more or less of fever with this complaint.

The symptoms attending piles are swellings at the verge of the anus, or in the rectum immediately above it, pain felt at the anus during the passage of the foeces, frequently an evacuation of blood, and occasional feelings of irritation in the parts affected. This disease is often preceded by other affections, such as giddiness of the head, difficulty of breathing, colicky pains, and pains in the loins.

The symptoms which attend the round worm of the intestines are a swelled belly, emaciated extremities, an offensive breath, and a deranged appetite. The appetite is often greater than in health, but sometimes it is much less. The stools are slimy; and the patient frequently picks his nose, and during sleep grinds his teeth.

Persons afflicted with the taenia complain of a gnawing uneasy feeling in the region of the stomach, which is removed, or diminished by eating. Their appetite is commonly somewhat voracious, but occasionally it is less than natural. They have commonly an itching at the nose, often nausea, colicky pains, and sometimes giddiness. Some have a cough, and other occasional convulsions.

When ascarides are lodged in the rectum, there is an uneasy feeling there, and a violent itching at the anus. There is also a sense of heat in the parts, with occasional tenemus and mucous stools. The mucus is sometimes mixed with blood, and along with it some living ascarides are often discharged (51).

When air is accumulated in a modern quantity in the bowels, it is known to exist by some fullness of the abdomen, and by the air shifting frequently its situation. This is sometimes attended with a kind of gurgling noise, and forms swellings in particular parts of the belly. A quantity of air is sometimes expelled by the mouth and the rectum. There is generally at the same time costiveness, and occasional colicky pains.

When air is accumulated in very large quantity, then it forms a very serious disease called tympanitis. Of this I have seen two or three instances. The belly is extremely swelled, with a very tense feeling, and there is a quick reaction of the parts after removing the pressure of the fingers from the belly, exactly similar to what takes place in a common ox's bladder, distended with air. This circumstance serves as one of the marks of distinction between tympanitis and ascites. There is no sense of fluctuation in tympanitis, but in ascites this is commonly distinct. There is often difficulty of breathing, which is produced by the accumulation of the air pushing up the diaphragm, and impeding its free motion.

---

51. See Med. Trans. of the College, Vol. I. p. 46.

There are severe colicky pains, and quantities of air are frequently expelled both upwards and downwards with a loud noise. The bowels are costive, and there is a difficulty in making water, which is probably occasioned by the accumulation of air in the rectum.

The symptoms of an inflamed mesentery cannot be separated from those which belong to inflammation of the peritonaeum generally; and these symptoms have been already described.

The symptoms which attend the enlargement of the mesenteric glands from scrofula correspond very much, in the most striking circumstances, with the symptoms which are produced by the common round worm of the intestines. In both diseases there is a tumid belly, and emaciated extremities. They are chiefly to be distinguished by worms not being discovered in the one disease, notwithstanding the use of strong purgatives, while they pass off from the bowels in the other. The startings, and the grinding of the teeth, may perhaps also form some ground of distinction between the two diseases: they occur very commonly in worms, but I believe rarely where the glands of the mesentery are scrofulous. Some discrimination likewise between the two diseases, may sometimes be derived from examining strictly into the nature of the constitution. If decided marks of scrofula shew themselves in an external part of the body, they will lead a practitioner more satisfactorily to the opinion that the mesenteric glands are also affected with the same disease.

CHAPTER IX

DISEASED APPEARANCES OF THE LIVER

Inflammation of the Membrane of the Liver

THE external membrane of the liver is not uncommonly found in a state of inflammation.

This may take place when the peritonaeum generally over the cavity of the abdomen is inflamed, or the inflammation may be confined to the membrane of the liver itself. When it is confined to the membrane of the liver, it is not frequently extended over the whole of it, but more commonly takes place in that part which covers the anterior, or convex part of the liver. I have also seen inflammation, or at least its effects, not infrequently on that side of the liver, which is in contact with the stomach and the duodenum.

When inflammation takes place in the membrane of the liver, it exhibits exactly the same appearances, which have been described when speaking of the inflammation of the peritonaeum, of which it is a part. It is crowded with a great number of very minute vessels, which contain florid blood, and is thicker than in its natural state. There is also thrown out upon its surface, a layer of coagulable lymph; this layer is thicker on some occasions than others, and often glues the liver, more or less completely to the neighbouring parts. Some quantity of serous fluid is at the same time thrown out.

Adhesions

It is more common to see adhesions formed, which are the consequence of a previous inflammation in the membrane of the liver, than to see the membrane in an actual state of inflammation. These adhesions are formed from the coagulable lymph of the blood, which undergoes a gradual progress of change, as we have formerly described. They consist very commonly of a thin, transparent membrane, which joins the surface of the liver to the neighbouring parts. This junction may either be general, over one extended surface of the liver, or it may consist of a number of processes of adhesion: the adhesion is sometimes by a membrane of considerable length; and sometimes the adhesion is very close, the surface of the liver being immediately applied to the neighbouring parts. The surface of the liver, where these adhesions are most commonly found, is the anterior, by which it is joined to the peritonaeum lining the muscles at the upper part of the cavity of the abdomen.

When an abscess is formed in the substance of the liver, and points externally, these adhesions are of great use in preventing the pus from escaping into the general cavity of the abdomen. Adhesions are also frequently found connecting the posterior surface of the liver to the stomach, and the duodenum; and these may also be useful in abscesses of the liver, near its posterior surface, by preventing the matter from passing into the general cavity of the abdomen, and conducting it either into the stomach, or the upper part of the intestinal canal.

Coats of the Liver converted into Cartilage

A part of the coats of the liver is sometimes changed into cartilage. Of this I have seen a few instances; but it occurs much more rarely in the liver than in the spleen. The cartilage is smooth and thin, and very soft in its texture.

Inflammation of the Substance of the Liver

It does not often happen, in this country, that the substance of the liver is found in an actual state of inflammation. Where its membrane is inflamed, the substance is sometimes inflamed which lies immediately under it; but it rarely happens that the general mass of the liver is inflamed. In warmer countries, the substance of the liver is much more liable to inflammation than in Great Britain. When the liver is generally inflamed through its substance, it is a good deal enlarged in size, and of a purple colour (52). It is also harder to the touch, than in its healthy state. Its outer membrane is sometimes affected by the inflammation, and sometimes it is not. It is attended occasionally with a jaundiced colour of skin, arising from the bile not getting readily into the ductus communis choledochus, on account of the pressure of the inflamed liver on the pori biliarii. When this inflammation has continued for some time, abscesses are formed, and then the active state of the inflammation very much subsides. These abscesses are sometimes of large size, so as even to contain some pints of pus. Sometimes the whole of the liver is almost converted into a bag containing pus. When inflammations of the liver have been of considerable standing, they are not uncommonly attended with ascites, and the water is of a yellow, or green colour, being tinged by the bile.

The liver has sometimes been said to have been in a state of mortification (53). This however occurs very rarely, and has never fallen under my own observation.

Common Tubercle of the Liver

One of the most common diseases in the liver (and perhaps the most common, except the adhesions which we have lately described,) is the formation of tubercles in its substance. This disease is hardly ever met with in a very young person, but frequently takes place in persons of middle or advanced age: it is likewise more common in men than women. This seems to depend upon the habit of drinking being more common in the one sex than in the other; for this disease is most frequently found in hard drinkers, although we cannot see any necessary connection between that mode of life and this particular disease in the liver. It happens, however, very commonly, that we can see little connection between cause and effect, in changes which are going on in

---

52. May not the purple arise from the accumulation of blood in the branches of the vena portarum?

As this vein performs the office of an artery in the liver, is it not probable that its small branches take on the same actions as the small branches of the artery during inflammation?

53. Vid. Morgagni Epist. XXXIV. Art. 25.

every other part of the body.

The tubercles which are formed in this disease occupy generally the whole mass of the liver, are placed very near each other, and are of a rounded shape; they give an appearance every where of irregularity to its surface. When cut into, they are found to consist of a brownish or yellowish white solid matter. They are sometimes of a very small size, so as not to be larger than the heads of large pins, but most frequently they are as large as small hazel nuts, and many of them are sometimes larger. When the liver is thus tuberculated, it feels much harder to the touch than natural, and not uncommonly its lower edge is bent a little forward. Its size, however, is generally not larger than in a healthy state, and I think it is often smaller. If a section of the liver be made in this state, its vessels seem to have a smaller diameter than they have naturally. It very frequently happens that in this state the liver is of a yellow colour, arising from the bile accumulated in its substance; and there is also water in the cavity of the abdomen, which is yellow from the mixture of bile. The gall-bladder is generally much contracted, and of a white colour, from its being empty. The bile, from the pressure of the hard liver upon the pori biliarii, does not reach the ductus hepaticus, and therefore cannot pass into the gall-bladder. The colour of the skin in such cases is jaundiced, and it remains permanently so, as it depends on a state of liver not liable to change. This is the common appearance of what is generally called a schirrhus liver: but it bears only a remote resemblance to schirrhus, as it shews itself in other parts of the body. I should therefore be disposed to consider it as a peculiar disease affecting this viscus.

Large White Tubercle of the Liver

Hard white masses are sometimes formed in the liver. They are often as large as chestnut; but I have seen them both a good deal larger and smaller than this size. They are to be found near the surface of the liver in greater number, than near the middle of its substance: two or three frequently lie contiguous to each other, with a considerable portion of the liver, in a healthy state, interposed between them and a cluster of similar tubercles. They consist of a very firm, opaque, white substance and are generally somewhat depressed, or hallow, upon their outer surface. The liver in this disease is frequently a good deal enlarged beyond its natural size.

These tubercles appear to be first formed round the blood vessels of the liver, as is seen in making sections of a liver in this state. While the liver is under such circumstances of disease, there is sometimes water in the cavity of the abdomen, and at other times none; the liver is sometimes tinged in its colour, from the accumulation of bile, and sometimes the colour of its substance between the tubercles is perfectly natural.

The kind of tubercle which we have now described, is much more rare than the other, and resembles more the ordinary appearance of schirrhus in other parts of the body. In one or two instances of it, however, I have observed a thick sort of pus, resembling very much the pus from a scrofulous sore; and therefore I am rather disposed to think that this tubercle may be of a scrofulous nature.

Soft brown tubercles of the Liver

I have also seen in the liver a number of soft tumours, about the size of a walnut: they were principally situated at the surface of the liver, and consisted of a smooth, soft, brownish matter. This is a very rare appearance of disease: such tumours would by many be considered as scrofulous, but there is no strong evidence in support of this opinion; and there is certainly no resemblance between this sort of tumour, and either a scrofulous tubercle of the lungs, or a scrofulous absorbent gland. About its real nature nothing satisfactory is ascertained.

Scrofulous Tubercles of the Liver

Tubercles are occasionally found in the liver, which bear a strong resemblance to the tubercles of the lungs; but this is a very rare appearance of disease. They have the same size, the same structure, and the same feeling to the touch, but are a little browner in their colour. In the only instance which I have seen of this disease, the tubercles were generally dispersed through the substance of the liver at pretty regular distances, and did not render the surface of the liver irregular, as in the common sort of tubercle. From their appearance and structure I cannot hesitate to consider them as scrofulous.

Liver flaccid, with reddish Tumours

I have likewise seen the liver much more flaccid in its membrane than is natural, with reddish tumours, of considerable size, interspersed through it, which contained a thick sort of pus. I am inclined to consider this liver as scrofulous, because it was found in a person whose general constitution had strong marks of scrofula, and in whom also were found many scrofulous absorbent glands on examining the body.

Liver very soft in its Substance

The liver is not unusually found much more flaccid in its substance than natural, without any other appearance of disease. It feels upon such occasions nearly as soft as the spleen, and is commonly of a leaden colour. This change must arise from a process which takes place through its whole substance, and seems to be what Mr. Hunter has called the interstitial absorption. By this process is meant, the absorbents removing insensibly the very minute parts out of the general mass of any structure in an animal body without ulceration. This state of liver is very rarely, if ever, found in a very young person, and is most common in persons who are advanced in life.

Liver very hard in its Substance

There is a very contrary state of the liver, not at all unusual, viz. where it is much harder than natural, and when cut into, exhibits no peculiar structure. Upon the surface of these livers, there is not uncommonly a thready appearance of membrane, disposed somewhat in a radiated form, and the lower edge is bent a little forwards. This I believe to be the first step in the progress towards the formation of the common tuberculated liver. I have sometimes seen small tubercles formed upon a part of the surface of such a liver, which were exactly of the common sort. From this appearance, it is probable, that additional matter is deposited in the interstices, through the general mass of the liver, rendering it much harder, and that this matter, together perhaps with part of the ordinary structure of the liver, is converted into tubercles. This hardened state of the liver is sometimes accompanied with a beginning ascites, and sometimes is without it.

Hydatids

There is no gland in the human body in which hydatids are so frequently found as the liver, except the kidneys, where they are still more common (54). Hydatids of the liver are usually found in a cyst, which is frequently of considerable size, and is formed of very firm materials, so as to give to the touch almost the feeling of cartilage. The cyst, when cut into, is obviously laminated, and is much thicker in one liver than another. In some livers it is not thicker than a shilling, and in others, it is near a quarter of an inch in thickness. The laminae which compose it are formed of a white-matter, and on the inside there is a lining of a pulpy substance, like the coagulable lymph. The cavity of the cyst I have seen, in one instance, subdivided by a partition of this pulpy substance. In a cyst may be found one hydatid, or a greater number of them. They lie loose in the cavity, swimming in a fluid; or some of them are attached to the side of the cyst. They consist of a round bag, which is composed of a white, semi-opaque, pulpy matter, and contain a fluid capable of coagulation. Although the common colour of hydatids be white, yet I have occasionally seen some of a light amber colour. The bag of the hydatid consists of two laminae, and possesses a good deal of contractile power. In one hydatid this coat, or bag, is much thicker and more opaque than in another, and even in the same hydatid different parts of it will often differ in its thickness. On the inside of an hydatid,

54. Although the hydatids of the liver, and the kidney, have got the same name, yet most frequently they differ from each other. Hydatids, however, occasionally occur in the kidneys, which are precisely of the same kind with those of the liver.

smaller ones are sometimes found which are commonly not larger than the heads of pins, but sometimes they are even larger in their size than a gooseberry. These are attached to the larger hydatid, either at scattered, irregular distances, or so as to form small clusters: and they are also found floating loose in the liquor of the larger hydatids. Hydatids of the liver are often found unconnected with each other; but sometimes they have been said to inclose each other in a series, like pill-boxes. The most common situation of hydatids of the liver, is in its substance, and inclosed in a cyst; but they are occasionally attached to the outer surface of the liver, hanging from it, and occupying more or less of the general cavity of the abdomen.

The origin and real nature of these hydatids are not fully ascertained; it is extremely probable, however, that they are a sort of imperfect animalcules. There is no doubt, that the hydatids in the livers of sheep are animalcules: they have been often seen to move when taken out of the liver, and put into warm water, and they retain this power of motion, for a good many hours after a sheep has been killed. The analogy is great between hydatids in the liver of a sheep, and in that of the human subject. In both they are contained in strong cysts, and in both they consist of the same white pulpy matter. There is undoubtedly some difference between them in simplicity of organization; the hydatid in the human liver being a simple uniform bag, and the hydatid in that of the sheep having a neck and mouth appended to the bag. This difference need be no considerable objection to the opinion above stated. Life may be attached to the most simple form of organization. In proof of this, hydatids have been found in the brains of sheep, resembling almost exactly those in the human liver, and which have been seen to move, and therefore are certainly known to be animalcules. The hydatids of the human liver indeed, have not as far as I know, been found to move when taken out of the body and put into warm water; had this ever happened, no uncertainty would remain. It is not difficult to see a good reason why there will hardly occur any proper opportunity of making this experiment. Hydatids are not very often found in the liver: and the body is allowed to remain for so long a time after death before it is examined, that the hydatids must have lost their living principle, even if they were animalcules. The probability of their being animalcules, however, is very strong; and it appears even more difficult to account for their production according to the common theory of generation, than for that of intestinal worms. We do not get rid of the difficulty by asserting, that hydatids in the human liver are not living animals, because in sheep they are certainly such, where the difficulty of accounting for their production is precisely the same. If any person should wish to consider hydatids more minutely, he will find an excellent account of them published by Dr. John Hunter in the Medical and Chirurgical Transactions (55).

Cysts in the Liver containing an Earthy Matter

Cysts are occasionally formed in the liver containing an earthy matter. The cysts are composed of a kind of cartilaginous substance mixed with bone. The earthy substance contained in the cyst is soft, smooth, and of a brownish white colour. It is mixed with soft films, resembling a good deal in their appearance the coats of a hydatid.

Rupture of the Liver

The liver is more liable to be ruptured by external violence than any other gland of the body, which probably arises from two causes: the one is, that in thin persons the liver, more especially when large, lies near the surface of the body, and therefore may be readily affected by a strong external pressure. The other is, that the liver consists of a structure, the parts of which are more easily separated from each other by pressure, than those of almost any other organ or structure in the body. Thus, if the thumb or the finger be pressed against the liver with a good deal of force, the liver gives way much in the same manner as a rotten pear would do, although not so readily. In this trial the effect does not depend upon the liver being softened by putrefaction, because it will take place in the liver of a person immediately after death. It depends

---

55. See Med. and Chirurgical Trans. p. 34.

upon the peculiar structure of the liver, and therefore may take place in the liver of a person, who is alive, as well as of one who is dead. If the same degree of pressure be applied to a muscle, or many glands of the body, they are not ruptured, but recover themselves after the pressure has been removed. When ruptures have taken place in the liver, they have happened from some strong pressure applied to the upper part of the abdomen; as for instance, from the wheel of a carriage passing over that part of the body. Little pain has been felt from such an injury; which is a proof among many others of the liver not possessing much sensibility; and some of the persons to whom this accident has happened have continued to live after it for several days.

Worms said to be in the Liver

Worms (56) have been said to be found in cysts of the liver, as well as in the biliary ducts. Instances of this sort are extremely rare, and have not come under my own observation.

SYMPTOMS

When the coats of the liver are inflamed, more especially upon its convex surface, the symptoms correspond a good deal with those of pleurisy, in which the inflammation has attacked the lower part of the pleura upon the right side. There is acute pain in the part affected, difficulty of breathing, cough, and symptomatic fever. The two affections may however, be in general, distinguished from each other by the following circumstances. Where the coats of the liver are inflamed the pain will be less increased upon deep inspiration than where the pleura at the lower part of the right side of the chest is inflamed. In inflammation of the coats of the liver there will be a considerable increase of pain upon pressure immediately under the margin of the ribs on the right side, which will not take place in inflammation of the pleura.

I am not acquainted with any symptoms which attend adhesions of the liver to the neighbouring parts.

---

56. Vid. Lieutaud, Tom. I. p. 194.

When the substance of the liver is inflamed, there is an obtuse pain in the right hypochondrium, and a pain is often felt at the top of the right shoulder. The patient can lie most easily on the side affected. There is more or less of symptomatic fever, sometimes a dry cough, sometimes hickup, sometimes vomiting, and occasionally a yellow colour of the skin and eyes. Inflammation of the substance of the liver sometimes takes place so very slowly, that it is hardly attended with any pain, and the constitution is not at all or very little affected with symptoms of fever. On such occasions an inflammation of the liver is not suspected till an abscess has actually been formed, and begins to make its progress outwards.

I know of no peculiar symptoms by which the liver can be ascertained, in the living body, to be studded with tubercles. When, however, there is pain or an uneasy feeling in the region of the liver, together with a jaundiced colour of the skin, which continues permanent, and water is at the same time accumulated in the cavity of the abdomen; there remains little doubt of the liver being tuberculated. When the parietes of the abdomen are thin, and water is accumulated in small quantity in that cavity, the tubercles at the lower edge of the liver can sometimes be distinctly felt by the fingers, upon an attentive examination.

The symptoms which belong to the large white tubercle of the liver, I cannot distinguish from those of the common tubercle. Sometimes, however, when the person is thin and the tubercles are near the lower edge of the liver, they can be distinguished by an external examination. I believe that the large white tubercle is not so often attended with jaundice and ascites as the other.

The symptoms which belong to the other tubercles of the liver are unknown to me. I am disposed to think that there are none which may be called discriminative.

When the liver is becoming hard in its substance, the exact state of it cannot be determined in the living body, unless the person be so thin that the liver can be distinctly felt upon examination. This, however, will frequently be very difficult, and on many occasions impossible; because the liver, when hard, is commonly not increased in its size, and the parietes of the abdomen are of considerable thickness. If there be some sense of uneasiness in the region of the liver, along with a sallow countenance, this disease may be suspected. It has sometimes happened, however, that the liver has been discovered to be hard, upon examination after death, when no symptoms had been observed during life, which led to an opinion of this disease having taken place.

There are no symptoms which characterize, particularly, the formation of hydatids in the liver, and this disease can only be guessed at in the living body. It appears from the history of some cases of this kind, that a pain is felt in the right hypochondrium; but this may arise from many other causes.

In two cases which have come to my knowledge the symptoms were similar to those which attend an attack of gall-stones. There was a violent spasmodic pain near the pit of the stomach, frequent vomiting, and jaundice, with a pulse not accelerated. These attacks occurred frequently in both cases after considerable intervals of tolerably good health.

When hydatids are confined within the substance of the liver, I do not see how it is possible that their existence should be ascertained; but when they are formed on the outer surface of the liver, near its lower edge, their existence may in some degree be ascertained by examination, more especially if the person be thin. When, however, the parietes of the abdomen are thick, and the hydatids, or their cysts are not distinct, but lie in contact with each other, making an irregular tumour, it will hardly be possible to form an accurate opinion by an examination. If the tumour be formed gradually, and the general health be little affected, it is probable that it consists of hydatids. An accurate attention to the feeling, which the tumour yields upon pressure, or upon striking it gently with the hand, may also assist in forming a probable conjecture about its nature. Where the tumour consists of hydatids, it will generally feel to a certain degree soft; and if the hydatids should be very large, there will probably be an obscure sense of fluctuation upon striking the tumour with one hand, while the other is applied to the opposite side of it. If moreover, the tumour should occupy a great part of the cavity of the abdomen, and can be clearly traced from the liver, as the source of its growth, there can be little doubt of the existence of hydatids under these circumstances.

CHAPTER X

DISEASED APPEARANCES IN THE GALL-BLADDER

Inflammation of its Coats

THE coats of the gall-bladder are very rarely inflamed, without inflammation of the membrane which covers the posterior surface of the liver. When inflammation attacks this membrane, it naturally spreads over the outer coat of the gall-bladder, which is a continuation of it, and may affect the other coats of the gall-bladder, if it should have arisen to a violent degree. Inflammation, however, of the outer coat of the gall-bladder will not commonly be attended with inflammation of the others, because it is not closely applied to them, there being interposed a considerable quantity of cellular membrane. The appearances of inflammation in the coats of the gall-bladder are similar to what take place in the inflammation of the stomach or intestines. These have been already fully described and need not be repeated.

Adhesions

It is a very common appearance, upon dissection, to find the gall-bladder connected by adhesions, either to the small end of the stomach, or the beginning of the duodenum. These are the consequence of a previous inflammation in the outer coat of the gall-bladder, and resemble exactly the adhesions which we have already described.

Ulcers in the Gall-Bladder

It is rare that inflammation of the gall-bladder advances to ulceration: the accumulation of gall-stones in it, as far as I have observed, rarely produces this effect (57). Ulceration of the gall-bladder, however, occasionally takes place, and I believe almost always begins in the inner membrane. Of this I have known two cases. In the one case, several ulcers were found in the inner membrane of the gall-bladder, while the other coats were not affected; and in the other there was one ulcer which had destroyed a part of all the coats.

Coats of the Gall-bladder thickened and hard Tubercles formed in them

I have only had an opportunity once of observing this change in the gall-bladder. Its coats were above a quarter of an inch thick, and were studded with tubercles of a considerable size, and very firm in their texture. The liver to which this gall-bladder belonged was affected with the same disease.

Coats of the Gall-bladder bony

I have likewise seen the coats of the gall-bladder very much thickened, and converted in many parts into a sort of bony substance; but this is to be considered as a very rare appearance of disease.

Diseased state of the Biliary Ducts—Their Dilatation

The most common diseased appearance of the biliary ducts is their dilatation. The ductus hepaticus, ductus cysticus, and ductus communis choledochus, are sometimes dilated to an almost incredible size. I have seen the ductus hepaticus and choledochus so much dilated as to be nearly an inch in the transverse diameter. These dilatations of the biliary ducts take place in consequence of the passage of gall-stones; and it is astonishing how large gall-stones sometimes are, which have been known to pass into the duodenum. This ought to afford a strong ground of comfort to persons who are labouring under this complaint.

57. Dr. Soemmerring, however, has seen a good many instances of ulcers in the inner surface of the gall-bladder, from the irritation of gall stones.

Obliteration of the Biliary Ducts

An obliteration of any of the biliary ducts happens very rarely, but instances of this disease have been discovered, and they may be traced to the following causes. One cause is a violent inflammation, which had taken place in the inner surface of some of the biliary ducts, and has terminated in an adhesion of its sides. This may be supposed to arise most commonly from the irritation of a rough gall-stone, in the passage towards the duodenum. A similar adhesion has been known to take place in other canals of the body, in consequence of violent inflammation there, as, for instance, in the vagina. Another cause, which may act upon the lower extremity of the ductus communis choledochus, obliterating its cavity at that part, is a violent inflammation of the duodenum at the entrance of the duct; the extremity of the duct being involved in the inflammation may have its canal obliterated. To this may be added, as a third cause of obliteration, a scirrhus, or any other enlargement of the round head of the pancreas, which may so press upon the lower extremity of the ductus communis choledochus, as to annihilate its cavity. It has only occurred to myself to have seen an instance of obliteration in the ductus cysticus; but Dr. Storer, of Nottingham, whose ability and industry in his profession are well known, has favoured me with an account of two cases of obliteration at the end of the ductus communis choledochus.

A preternatural Canal of Communication between the Gall-bladder and the Stomach

It may not be improper to take notice here, that I have once seen an immediate communication, but a short canal between the gall-bladder and the small end of the stomach. This lusus naturae is very rare, and but a few instances of it have been recorded.

Gall-stones

It is not an uncommon appearance of disease in examining dead bodies, to find gall-stones, either in the gall-bladder, or in some of the biliary ducts. The gall-bladder is sometimes much enlarged in its size, and full of them. In this case its coats are often a good deal thickened, which arises partly from the pressure against the gall-bladder, in consequence of the accumulation of the stones, and partly from the efforts of the contractile power of the gall-bladder to expel them. The number of stones accumulated in the gall-bladder is sometimes very great; above a thousand have been taken out of one gall-bladder, which are preserved in Dr. Hunter's collection. When there is a solitary gall-stone in the gall-bladder, it is occasionally very large; I have known an instance of one which was fully the size of a hen's egg. When there is but one gall-stone either in the gall-bladder, or in the biliary ducts, it is generally of an oval shape; when there is a considerable number, they acquire, by rubbing upon each other, in a small space, a great many sides and angles.

There is great variety in the external appearance of gall-stones as to colour: some are whitish, others are black; they are also of a yellowish, a greenish, a light brown, a dark brown, and a reddish brown colour. These are the principal varieties in colour, but there are many other smaller differences which it is very difficult to express in words. Gall-stones differ also very much in the state of their surface, some being very smooth, and others a good deal roughened.

When cut or broken, gall-stones are commonly found to consist of concentric laminae upon the outside, and in the centre of a radiated structure. The laminated part bears sometimes a great proportion to the other, and sometimes the contrary happens. The laminated and radiated structures are sometimes compact, and sometimes consist of a more loose matter. It likewise occasionally happens that both the laminated and the radiated structures are very obscure, and the gall-stone appears a good deal like an uniform solid mass. The laminated part on the outside very frequently consists of a different substance, in appearance, from the radiated structure in the centre; and it is not unusual to find the structure in the centre to consist of shining, white crystallizations, which have a good deal the look of mica or spermaceti.

Gall-stones being very different both in their outward appearance and their internal structure from each other, we are naturally led to suppose that they may also differ in their chemical properties. Upon this subject I can only speak very generally; but such trials as I have made incline me to this opinion. Very few gall-stones yield a bitter taste, which shews that commonly they do not consist of inspissated bile; but in some I have found the taste intensely bitter. Almost all of them melt in the flame of a candle; but I have met with one sort, of a very black colour, which did not melt, but burnt exactly like a cinder (58).

All the gall-stones which I have examined dissolve in the nitrous acid. They are separated into a fine black powder when put into the vitriolic acid, especially if exposed to a sand heat. By the marine acid they are not acted upon at all in the common heat of the atmosphere; and are even but little affected by it when exposed to a sand heat for a considerable time.

Most of the gall-stones which I have examined, are either not very soluble in oil of turpentine, in the common heat of the atmosphere, or the process goes on very slowly: one sort I have found to be in this heat altogether insoluble. When put into this oil, and exposed to a sand heat, they are much more readily acted upon. Some are converted into a kind of oil, which sinks to the bottom of the oil of turpentine; others are partly soluble, tinging the oil of turpentine of a brownish colour, and are partly separated into a powder.

Most gall-stones appear not to be readily affected by the spirit of wine in the common heat of the atmosphere, but are either partly or entirely soluble in it in a boiling heat (59). Such are the general results from a good many trials of my own, but I should rest upon them with little confidence, if they did not in great measure correspond with those of the experiments of others, who

---

58. Dr. Soemmerring considers these as inspissated bile, and mentions, that they have no regular form, have a bitter taste, and are soluble in water. In some trials which I made they did not dissolve in distilled water, either cold or hot; but they are bitter to the taste, and without any regular shape, or appearance of crystallization.

59. When some biliary calculi are exposed to spirit of wine in a boiling state, white flaky crystals are soon formed upon its cooling. When they are exposed to spirit of wine in the common heat of the atmosphere, it is some weeks before crystals begin to be formed, and they appear to be more pointed in their shape than the former. These crystals were, I believe, first observed by M. Poullerier de la Salle. See Elements d'Histoire Naturalle et de Chimie, p i M. de Fourcroy, Tom. IV. p. 354.

are more conversant than myself both with the scientific and practical part of chemistry.

Gall-stones, according to the experiments of Gren, consist of a substance possessing the properties of wax, and of lymph (60).

A gall-stone, consisting of a chocolate coloured substance on the outside, and of white, radiated laminae upon the inside, was found by Dr. Saunders to consist of a resinous matter, with a small proportion of earth, apparently the calcareous, and some mineral and volatile alkali (61).

The gall-stones which Dr. Powell examined were found to consist of resinous matter, carbone, and an animal substance resembling dried mucus (62). This subject seems still to be imperfectly known, and to require further investigation.

Bile

The bile in the gall-bladder is found to differ in different bodies; but this is too common to arise from disease, and must depend on natural circumstances. It is sometimes of a green, at other times of a brownish yellow, or a purer yellow colour. The brownish yellow colour is the most common. It is always more or less viscid, and the variety in this respect is considerable: in man it generally appears a good deal more viscid than in most other classes of animals. In one case, I have seen it as ropy as the mucus which is commonly coughed up from the trachea. I recollect also another case, where the bile in the gall-bladder resembled exactly the white of a raw egg. This kind of substance is ascertained to form one of the constituent parts of the bile, and in the present instance it would seem that the other parts were wanting. Such an effect may be supposed to have depended upon a very imperfect action of the secretory structure of the liver. The liver was not sound, being studded with scrofulous tubercles, and the absorbent glands of the mesentery were affected with the same disease.

In opening dead bodies, the bile is almost always found to have transuded in small quantity through coats of the gall-bladder, so as to tinge the neighbouring parts, especially the small end of the

60. See Johnson's Animal Chemistry, Vol. 2, p. 355.
61. See Dr. Saunder's Treatise on the Liver, p. 119, first edition.
62. See Dr. Powell's Observations on the Bile and its disease.

stomach and the beginning of the duodenum. This is to be considered as a natural effect, which has taken place after death, and not as a diseased appearance. The coats of the gall-bladder, in consequence of death, have lost that compactness by which they were formerly able to confine the bile; it therefore transudes in small quantity, and tinges the neighbouring parts.

Gall-Bladder distended with Bile

The gall-bladder is sometimes distended with bile so as to be of nearly twice its usual size; at other times there is no bile at all in its cavity, and under such circumstances it is white in its colour, and contracted into very small size.

Hydatids in the Gall-bladder

The gall-bladder has been known to be distended to an immense size, and to contain hydatids (63); but this state of it is to be considered as extremely uncommon.

The Gall-bladder wanting

The gall-bladder has also been known to be wanting from a defect in the original formation (64). It has never occurred to me to see an example of this kind of monstrosity; but it may be the more readily believed sometimes to happen, as the gall-bladder does not serve any necessary purpose in the body. There are many classes of animals which are naturally without a gall-bladder.

SYMPTOMS

Inflammation of the coats of the gall-bladder is not known to be distinguished by any peculiar symptoms. They are probably much the same with the symptoms which attend inflammation of the membranous covering of the liver.

An obliteration either of the hepatic duct, or of the ductus communis choledochus, must produce a jaundice which is

63. See Medical Communications, Vol. I. p. 101.
64. See Dr. Soemmerring's Germ. Trans. p. 159.

permanent, because it depends upon a cause not liable to change. This will be extremely difficult to distinguish, in practice, from jaundice produced by a hardened, or tuberculated state of the liver, for this cause of jaundice may likewise be said to be generally permanent. When the ductus cysticus only is obliterated, there will be no jaundice, and little inconvenience will probably be felt, unless the bile confined in the gall-bladder should at length irritate its coats. In this case inflammation may be excited, which may advance to suppuration. I have seen an ulcer of the gall-bladder, which appeared to be produced by this cause.

While gall-stones remain in the gall-bladder, and no attempt is made towards their passing through the ductus cysticus, and ductus communis choledochus, very little inconvenience is commonly produced by them. It frequently happens that gall-stones are found in the gall-bladder after death, where there was not the least suspicion of their existence during life. When they pass through the ducts, more especially if they be large in their size, a most extruciating pain is commonly felt about the pit of the stomach: patients in this case express a much stronger feeling of pain, than during a violent inflammation even in the most sensible parts of the body. They often cry out, and writhe or twist their body into various postures. When the pulse is felt during this exquisite pain, it is sometimes found to be accelerated in a very trifling degree, but generally it is not more frequent than in health, and sometimes it is even slower. There is languor, sickness, and vomiting: and the skin becomes in the progress of the disease more or less of a yellow colour.

CHAPTER XI

DISEASED APPEARANCES OF THE SPLEEN

Inflammation of the Coats of the Spleen

THE coats of the spleen are liable to inflammation; but this rarely takes place unless the peritonaeum in the neighborhood be also affected. The proper capsule of the spleen is so intimately connected with the peritonaeum which is reflected over it, that it must necessarily partake of any inflammation, affecting that portion of the membrane. When inflammation attacks the coats of the spleen, it exhibits exactly the same appearances which have been so often described. They become much more crowded with florid blood vessels than in a natural state, are somewhat thicker, and throw out a layer of coagulable lymph upon their surface.

Adhesions

It is more common, however, to find adhesions formed between the spleen and the neighbouring parts, than to find its coats in an actual state of inflammation. These adhesions consist of a white, transparent membrane, of more or less firmness, and generally connect the broad surface of the spleen more or less closely to the diaphragm. They often connect too the spleen to the great end of the stomach, and a part of the transverse arch of the colon.

Inflammation of the substance of the Spleen

It is very rare to find the substance of the spleen either in a state of inflammation or suppuration; but such cases have occasionally been observed and related by authors (65). Instances

65. Vid. Li eutaud, Tom. I. p. 222.

also have been related where the spleen had been observed to be mortified (66); but this is probably much more rare than the former.

The Spleen extremely soft

There is an appearance of the spleen which is very common, and which perhaps is hardly to be considered as a disease, but it is a very obvious deviation from its healthy structure. The appearance to which I allude is an extreme softness of the spleen, so that when its capsule is broken (which under such circumstances is very tender) the substance of the spleen seems to consist of little else than a very soft, brownish red mucus, intermixed with a spongy fibrous texture. This appearance of the spleen is hardly ever to be observed at a very early period of life, but is very common in middle and more advanced age. I believe that such a state of the spleen is not marked by any peculiar feelings, so as to make the persons conscious of any disease taking place, and is probably of very little consequence in the general economy of the animal. Still, however, it is not a state into which the spleen naturally degenerates in the gradual decay of the body.

The Spleen very hard

The spleen is sometimes much harder than natural, and at the same time is generally a good deal enlarged. It will occasionally be enlarged to five or six times its natural size, and it then forms a tumour, very capable of being distinguished by an examination in the living body. When cut into, the natural structure seems to be preserved, except that it is much more compact, the parts being much more closely applied together.

This state of the spleen is generally considered as scirrhus; but its structure is not similar to scirrhus in other parts of the body; and its real nature is probably at present not fully understood. When the spleen is in this state, water is sometimes accumulated in the cavity of the abdomen.

---

66. Vid. Lieutaud, Tom. I. 223.

Tubercles in the Spleen

The spleen is sometimes, although rarely, studded in its substance with small tubercles, very similar to the scrofulous tubercles of the lungs. In one instance I have seen some of these in a state of suppuration, and the pus was thick and curdly, like scrofulous pus.

Coats of the Spleen Cartilaginous

The coats of the spleen are sometimes converted into cartilage; and this disease may be considered in a great measure as peculiar to the spleen. It is, at least, much more common in this viscus than in any other.

The cartilage is generally to be found on the convex surface of the spleen, and extends over more or less of it, in different cases. It is much thicker in one case than another: in some being no thicker than a shilling, and in others being four times as thick. It is generally formed in a smooth layer, but occasionally it is somewhat irregular. I have also seen, in some instances, small spots of cartilage over the whole surface of the spleen. It would appear that ossifications (67) are sometimes to be found in this cartilage, but in the cases which have come under my own examination, bony matter was not to be observed. The cartilage into which the coats of the spleen are changed, does not resemble the cartilage at the extremities of the bones, but more that of the nose and ears, although it is generally of a whiter colour. This diseased process, it is natural to think, is slow in its progress, can hardly produce any impediment to the functions of the spleen, and is probably not marked by any peculiar feelings to the patient.

Spleen very large

The spleen is sometimes found to be much larger in its size than natural, but with a structure perfectly healthy; and this more commonly happens to the spleen than to any other viscus.

67. Morgagni has seen ossification of a part of the capsule of the spleen. Vid. Epist. X. Art. 19. Epist. XIV. Art. 23.

Although it may be looked upon as a monstrous growth of the spleen, rather than a disease, yet it may produce inconvenience by its pressure, and by altering in some degree the situation of the neighbouring viscera.

Hydatids in the Spleen

Hydatids are occasionally found in the spleen (68), which are of the same kind with those of the liver; but they are much more common in the latter viscus, than in the former.

Stony Concretions in the Spleen

Stony concretions (69) have been seen occasionally in the spleen; but such cases are very rare, and have not fallen under my own observation.

The Spleen ruptured

The spleen has been known sometimes to be ruptured, in consequence of external pressure upon that side of the body where it is situated. When the spleen is of the common size, an accident of this kind very rarely takes place, because it is well defended by the ribs of the left side; but when the spleen is very large, so that a part of it passes below the margin of the ribs into the cavity of the flank, such an accident may very readily happen.

Several small Spleens

There is a variety in the natural formation of the spleen, which I believe does not take place in that of any other gland in the body. It consists in several small spleens being formed besides the common one. They vary in size in different instances, but I have seen some of them as large as a walnut. They are situated in the omentum, near the great end of the stomach, are supplied with blood vessels from the splenic artery and vein, and have exactly

68. Vid. Morgagni, Epist. XXXVIII. Art. 34.
69. Vid. Lieutaud, Tom. I. p. 231.

the same structure as a common spleen. It will probably make no difference with regard to the use of the spleen, whether it be entirely formed of one mass, or whether it consists of several distinct parts.

Spleen said to be wanting

The spleen has been said to be occasionally wanting, as a defect in the natural formation, but this too is very uncommon (70). We know that an animal is capable not only of existing, but also of enjoying good health without a spleen. The spleen has been cut out by way of experiment, from some quadrupeds, and they did not appear to suffer any inconvenience from the want of it. The human spleen has even been removed in a few instances, and the persons have not only recovered, but have enjoyed afterwards good health. It does not appear, therefore, very wonderful that a body should be formed without a spleen, and carry on its vital functions without any obvious imperfection.

SYMPTOMS

When inflammation attacks the coats of the spleen, it is attended with the same symptoms as an inflammation of that portion of the peritonaeum, which lies in the left hypochondrium. There is pain in that region, which is more or less acute according to the degree of the inflammation; and this pain is increased upon pressure. If the inflammation be considerable, it is accompanied with symptomatic fever.

The symptoms which have been described as belonging to inflammation of the substance of the spleen, are a fullness and sense of pain in the left hypochondrium. The pain is increased upon pressure, and there is more or less of symptomatic fever. In two cases of inflamed spleen, examined by the late Dr. Hunter, where the inflammation had advanced to suppuration, the patients could not define accurately the seat of their pain, but the pain seemed to travel a good deal over the general cavity of the abdomen.

---

70. Vid. Lieutaud, Tom. I. p. 234.

An enlarged and hardened state of the spleen is not suspected or known till the disease has made a considerable progress, so that the spleen is capable of being felt externally. It is commonly attended with no pain, and will even bear a pretty strong pressure, without any painful sensation. It may be distinguished when the spleen has arrived at a considerable size, by the situation and the general shape of the tumour. The anterior edge of the spleen can generally be felt distinctly by the hand applied to the surface of the abdomen, under the margin of the ribs upon the left side; and the edge is sometimes distinguished by this examination to be notched. This state of the spleen is often at length attended with dropsy.

There are no peculiar symptoms which characterize the formation of hydatids in the spleen. A pain has been remarked to be felt, in such cases, in the left hypochondrium, but this also belongs to many other complaints. When a swelling begins in the situation of the spleen, and spreads very slowly into the cavity of the abdomen, being somewhat soft to the feeling, and perhaps giving some obscure sense of fluctuation, the disease may then be reasonably supposed to depend on the formation of hydatids in this organ.

CHAPTER XII

DISEASED APPEARANCES OF THE PANCREAS

THE pancreas is subject to very few diseases. It seldom happens, upon examining dead bodies, that it exhibits any other than the healthy structure.

Abscess of the Pancreas

Inflammation is very little apt to affect the pancreas. It has only occurred to me to see one instance of an abscess formed in it. It was a good deal enlarged in its size, and contained a considerable quantity of thin pus.

Pancreas hard

It is not very uncommon to find the pancreas much harder than in its natural state, and at the same time it is thicker and shorter than usual. There is, however, little appearance to the eye of its structure being altered. This I believe to be the beginning of a process, by which the pancreas becomes truly schirrhus. It very seldom in this state shews, in any part, the real schirrhus structure. But I have seen this to be the case, which renders it very probable, that the one is the beginning of a change into the other. When the pancreas in any part assumes the schirrhus structure, that part loses entirely its natural appearance, and is converted into a hard, uniform, white mass, somewhat intersected by membrane, like schirrhus in other parts of the body. In some cases it has been observed, in this state, to be considerably enlarged.

Calculi of the Pancreas

Calculi are occasionally formed in the ducts of the pancreas. Of this I have known only one instance. The calculi were about the size of the kernel of a hazle nut, with a very irregular surface, and of a white colour. These stones dissolved in marine acid with the extraction of a large quantity of carbonic gas and are found to consist of carbonated lime (71). It is not improbable, that calculi formed in the pancreas may differ somewhat from each other, as we find to happen in other calculi which are formed in the body; but as this is a very rare disease in the pancreas, it must be a long time before this point can be fully ascertained.

Pancreas wanting

The pancreas has been said to be entirely wanting, as a defect in the original formation (72).

SYMPTOMS

I have only had one opportunity of seeing an abscess in the pancreas. It was in a young man, a little beyond the age of twenty. He did not complain of any fixed pain in the situation of the pancreas, but had a good deal of pain in different parts of the abdomen. This seemed to be connected with spasmodic contractions of the intestinal canal, which inclosed portions of wind, and also with spasms of the abdominal muscles. There was sickness and distention of the stomach more especially after eating, and the food likewise sometimes occasioned a sense of weight in that organ. He had a disposition to purging; made but little water; and became at length dropsical. His pulse was commonly about eighty (73). Some cases which are related in books, I find that patients with abscesses in the pancreas have commonly complained of pain in the back and loins, but they seem to have had no peculiar symptoms.

When the pancreas becomes harder than in its healthy state, it is often, I believe, not attended with any painful sensations to the

---

71. See Dr. Pemberton's Treatise upon the Abdominal Viscera, p. 92.
72. Vid. Lieutaud, Tom. I. p. 247.
73. For the account of the symptoms in the above case, I am indebted to Dr. Wm. Herberden.

patient which are strongly marked. But it sometimes happens, although rarely, that the pancreas becomes much enlarged in its size, as well as hard in its structure, undergoing these changes which belong to scirrhus. In such cases, a long continued pain has been remarked to exist in the epigastric region, and the stomach has been affected with sickness. In one instance, of which I have heard an account, besides the symptoms already mentioned, there was a pain in the hips, and a sense of numbness in one thigh and leg.

I am not acquainted with the symptoms which are produced by the formation of calculi in the pancreas. If the calculi should happen to be smooth, and few in number, they would probably occasion little pain or inconvenience. But if they should be rough upon their surface and numerous, they would probably produce a good deal of irritation and pain in the pancreas; but it is not likely that we should be able to guess at the cause of the irritation, unless some of the calculi having passed into the duodenum, should be evacuated by vomiting, or by stool.

CHAPTER XIII

DISEASED APPEARANCES OF THE KIDNEYS AND THE RENAL CAPSULES

Capsule of the Kidneys inflamed

I DO not recollect to have seen the proper capsule of the kidney inflamed, and I am disposed to consider it as a rare morbid appearance. The reason, probably, why it seldom occurs, is that the peritonaeum reflected over the surface of the kidney has a very loose connection with it, there being interposed between them a considerable quantity of cellular membrane and fat. It seems very likely that the principal reason why the capsules of some other glands in the abdomen are so frequently inflamed, is their close connection with the peritonaeum; which membrane, from circumstances it is perhaps difficult to ascertain, is very liable to inflammation. When the capsule of the kidneys is inflamed, the same appearances of inflammation will take place which have been so often noted.

Abscesses of the Kidneys

When the substance of the kidneys is inflamed, it frequently advances to suppuration, and perhaps there is no considerable gland in the body so liable to form abscesses as the kidneys. In some cases which I have seen, the abscesses have appeared to be of a common nature; but in the greater number of cases they have been scrofulous.

When a kidney is attacked with scrofula, and the disease has advanced to suppuration, it exhibits different appearances, according to the degree of the advancement. Sometimes there are only one or two circumscribed abscesses, containing a curdly pus, without anything being particularly observable in the inner surface of the abscesses. Frequently, however, the inner surface of the abscesses is lined with a pulpy matter. These abscesses generally first destroy the mamillary portion of the kidney; and when they advance very far, they destroy almost the whole structure of the kidney, converting it into capsules which surround a number of imperfect cavities that are lined with this pulpy substance.

The capsule into which a kidney is changed by the progress of this disease, is on some occasions thicker than on others, frequently of considerable hardness, and seems sometimes to be slightly laminated. When a kidney is so affected, it is not uncommon for the pelvis and ureter to partake of the disease, and a calculus is often found either in the abscess, or in the pelvis of the ureter (74).

Scrofulous Tubercles in the Kidneys

It is not unusual (as we have stated above) for scrofulous abscesses to take place in the kidneys, but it occurs very rarely that scrofulous tubercles are formed in them. I have seen, however, an instance of this kind, and the tubercles resembled most exactly the common tubercles of the lungs. None of them were in a state of suppuration.

Kidney Scirrhus

The kidney I have once seen converted into a firm, uniform substance, somewhat intersected by membrane, in which the natural structure of this gland was entirely lost. The kidney was at the same time very much enlarged in size. This alteration of structure I should call scirrhus, because it exactly resembles scirrhus in other parts of the body: it occurs very rarely in the kidneys.

State of the Kidneys in Diabetes

Opportunities do not frequently occur of examining the state of

---

74. In such cases, it is very probable that the calculus is the immediate cause of the other disease, the constitution being at the same time disposed to it. By the irritation of the calculus, inflammation and suppuration are produced in the kidney, and these partake of the nature of the constitution.

the kidneys in diabetes. I have once, however, been able to make this examination in a satisfactory manner, where a person had been long affected with diabetes, and had been a patient under my care at St. George's Hospital. In both kidneys the superficial veins were much fuller of blood than usual, forming upon their surface a most beautiful network of vessels. The whole substance of the kidneys was much more vascular than in a healthy state, approaching a good deal in appearance to what takes place in inflammation. In both of them there was a very small quantity of a whitish fluid, somewhat resembling pus; but there was no appearance of ulceration whatever. The artery, the vein, the lymphatic vessels, and the nerves of both kidneys were in their natural state. The liver, at the same time, I examined with care, because it has been thought by some to be the chief source of disease in diabetic patients, but it was perfectly sound. The stomach and intestines were also examined with attention, but no appearances occurred in them which are not very common.

Kidneys very soft

I have also seen the substance of the kidney converted into a soft loose mass, resembling almost exactly the appearance of common sponge. On the surface there were many round interstitial cavities scattered at irregular distances; and when the substance of the kidney was cut into, it exhibited the same spongy structure. The blood vessels of the kidney were seen ramifying very distinctly through the spongy mass. There was no appearance of pus in the kidney, nor was there the most distant resemblance between this process, and the effects produced by suppuration. It was a process of a peculiar kind, by which a considerable portion of the kidney was removed by the action, probably, of absorbent vessels, and it seemed to act much more on the cortical than the tubular part of it. I am not at all exaggerating the effect of this diseased process when I say, that the kidney was rendered fully as soft as a common sponge. When shaken in water, the parts all separated from each other, somewhat like the unravelling of the shaggy vessels of the placenta. Such an appearance of kidney, but in a much smaller degree, has fallen two or three times under my observation.

Hydatids of the Kidneys

The formation of hydatids is not an uncommon disease in the kidneys. There are sometimes one or two considerable hydatids on the surface of the kidney, lying between its substance and capsule; at other times, they are more numerous. These hydatids do not appear to be of the same nature with the hydatids of the liver: they are not inclosed in firm cysts; their coats are also thinner, and less pulpy; and not uncommonly they are almost as thin as any membrane of the body. I do not recollect to have seen any instance of small hydatids of this sort attached to the coats of larger hydatids in the kidney, as may be frequently observed in the liver. It is therefore probable, that the hydatids which are commonly found in the kidney, depend on a diseased alteration of the structure of this organ, and are not distinct organized simple animals.

Sometimes, however, the true hydatid is formed in the kidneys, having exactly the same nature with that which grows in the liver. It has occurred to me to be able to examine particularly a case of this kind after death, and I shall describe at some length what came under my observation. The right kidney, in a soldier, was converted into a bag capable of containing at least three pints of fluid, and only a very small part of the kidney at the lower end retained its natural structure. The bag was of considerable thickness, was obscurely laminated, and had a cartilaginous hardness upon its inner surface. It was full of hydatids, which differed very much from each other in their size, some of them being as large as a small orange, and others not larger than the head of a pin. Some of the small hydatids were lodged in little cavities formed in the inner surface of the bag. Their coats were in general easily separable into two laminae, and varied a good deal in thickness in different hydatids. This difference made one hydatid look opaque, while another was transparent. Even in the same hydatid there was often a difference in the opacity, or transparency of its coat at different parts. Some hydatids had, adhering to their inner surface, a cluster of small hydatids, which looked like small pearls; others had hydatids even of a considerable size floating loose in their cavity; and others contained only a fluid. The fluid in many was transparent, but in some hydatids it resembled whey. Some of the small hydatids had frequently been passed along with the urine, when the person was alive. It required an increased exertion of the muscular power of the bladder to drive them through the urethra, and the bladder, by this exertion acquired a stronger muscular coat, as in other cases of obstruction to the free passage of the urine.

Calculi of the Kidneys

The formation of calculi is not peculiar to the kidneys, but it is a more frequent disease in them than in any other part of the body. Small granules of stone are sometimes found in the tubular portion of the kidneys; but it is more common to find a calculus of considerable size lodged either in some part of the substance of the kidney, or in the pelvis of the ureter. The last situation is by much the most frequent. When a stone in this situation is so large as not to be capable of passing through the ureter, it is afterwards gradually increased in size, from the contact of the urine. In its growth, it necessarily follows the branches of the pelvis, which are called infundibula, and is therefore of an arborescent form. Such calculi vary in their colour and surface; they are sometimes of a light brown, sometimes of a dark brown, and sometimes of a white colour. They are also sometimes smooth, and sometimes a little roughened on their surface. Of the nature of urinary calculi we shall speak afterwards, when we come to take notice of the diseased appearances of the bladder. When a stone in the pelvis of the ureter has increased to a very considerable size, it almost entirely prevents the urine from passing into the ureter. The urine is therefore accumulated in the pelvis above the stone, and hence enlarges the pelvis very much, as well as the cavity in the kidney itself. From the pressure too of the urine behind the stone, the pelvis of the ureter, besides being enlarged, is thrust out from the substance of the kidney. If the interruption to the passage of the urine from the kidney arises from some obstruction in the lower extremity of the ureter, or at the neck of the bladder, or in any part of the urethra, not only the pelvis of the ureter is then enlarged, but the ureter itself. I have seen the ureters of both kidneys enlarged from this cause to twice or thrice their natural size.

Whatever be the nature of the obstruction, if the pelvis of the ureter be very much enlarged from the accumulation of the urine, the cavity of the kidney is at the same time enlarged. As this process advances, the substance of the kidney becomes more and more compressed, is gradually absorbed and its cavity becomes enlarged in proportion. The substance of the kidney is, at length, in a great measure lost, and is converted into a capsule, containing a great many cells, which communicate with each other. The capsule is sometimes very thin, and the whole mass a great deal larger than the natural size of a healthy kidney. It is worthy of remark, that the urine is secreted even when the natural structure of the kidney is almost entirely lost. This is seen both in the derangement of the kidneys now under consideration, and when they are converted into a mass of hydatids. It would appear from this fact, that a very small portion of the natural structure of the kidneys is capable of secreting very nearly the ordinary quantity of the urine.

Kidneys earthy and bony

The kidneys have been said to be converted into an earthy substance (75). A kidney has also been known to become ossified (76). Such appearances have never come under my own observation, and I am persuaded are extremely rare.

Original Varieties in the Kidneys

The kidneys are subject to a good deal of variety in their natural circumstances, from original formation. The two kidneys are sometimes found to be joined together: they are sometimes situated before the lumbar vertebrae, and sometimes on the sides of the pelvis. They are occasionally very small in their size, and the kidney on one side is sometimes wanting; when this is the case, the other kidney is larger than the ordinary size.

It is very difficult to assign a satisfactory reason why there should be such variety in the kidneys; but we can see that there is

75. Vid. Lieutaud, Tom. I. p. 282.
76. See Medical Communications, Vol. I. p. 416.

little disadvantage to the animal functions produced by this variety.

The kidneys are not large in their size, and therefore may be changed in their situation without any sensible inconvenience. As their function is independent of relative situation, it must be precisely the same wherever the kidneys are placed.

When the kidneys are small, the secretion of the urine may be very nearly in the common quantity, from a great activity in carrying on their function; or such persons may be disposed to sweat more than usual, to counterbalance the deficiency of the urine. We know very well that the secretions of the sweat and the urine are vicarious. When a kidney is wanting, the other being of a large size is probably capable of doing the office of two kidneys.

Diseased Appearances of the Renal Capsules

The renal capsules are scarcely ever found diseased. The dark coloured substance in their centre, which naturally has some consistence, is occasionally very soft, so as almost to be fluid. This is probably what is meant by authors, when they say that they have found in the cavity of the renal capsules a fluid like ink. Their description may be considered as being a little exaggerated.

Abscess in the Renal Capsules

The renal capsules are very seldom attached with inflammation, and therefore abscesses have very rarely occurred in them. There is much variety in the different parts of the body, with regard to their susceptibility of being excited to inflammation. A few cases of abscesses in the renal capsules are related by authors.

Renal Capsule scrofulous

It has occurred to me to see only one instance of scrofula in the renal capsules (77). In this case the renal capsule affected by it was very much enlarged in its size, being nearly as large as a kidney,

---

77. See Soemmerring's German Translation, p. 173.

and was changed into the same kind of white matter which is observable in a scrofulous absorbent gland.

The renal capsules have also been observed to be changed into a cartilaginous substance, but this morbid appearance occurs very rarely.

Little granules of stone have been found in the substance of the renal capsules (78).

SYMPTOMS

When the kidneys are inflamed, more or less pain is felt in the situation of these glands, and the pain commonly shoots along the course of the ureters. There is a sense of numbness in the thigh, and in the male there is often a retraction of the testicle, or a feeling of pain in it. When one kidney is affected, these symptoms are only felt upon that side. The urine is voided frequently, and sometimes of a pale, but more commonly of a deep red colour. The stomach sympathizes with this state of the kidneys, for it is affected with sickness and vomiting; the bowels are at the same time often costive, and subject to colicky pains. These sensations are accompanied with more or less of symptomatic fever.

When pus is formed by the progress of the inflammation, it may be known by its being mixed with the urine, and this will be more distinctly marked in proportion to the quality of the pus.

The symptoms which belong to a scirrhous state of the kidneys are unknown to me, and I do not find that they are distinctly marked by authors.

There would seem to be no particular symptoms which belong to the formation of hydatids in the kidneys. Pain is commonly felt in the loins during their formation; there has been remarked to be symptomatic fever, nausea, and vomiting; but these symptoms belong also to some other diseases. This disease, therefore, can only be ascertained by hydatids passing occasionally through the urethra along with the urine. In such cases, there must sometimes be a difficulty in making water, from a hydatid interrupting the passage of the urine, either at the neck of the bladder, or in some

78. Vid. Lieutaud, Tom. I. p. 286.

part of the urethra.

The symptoms which are produced by calculi irritating the kidneys correspond very much with the symptoms attending the inflammation of these organs. The irritation from calculi, however, may be distinguished from simple inflammation of the kidneys, by these additional symptoms, viz. by red crystals being often deposited from the urine as soon as it is voided, by blood being sometimes mixed with the urine, and by the pain of the loins being much increased upon any jolting motion of the body.

Diabetes is distinguished by the urine being much increased beyond the natural quantity, by its being more or less sweet to the taste, and of a colour somewhat resembling whey. There is great thirst, and a voracious appetite for food. The pulse is also somewhat quicker than natural, and the body becomes at length much emaciated.

CHAPTER XIV

DISEASED APPEARACES OF THE BLADDER

Inflammation of the Peritonaeal Covering

THAT portion of the peritonaeum, which covers a part of the bladder, is not very often inflamed by itself, but it partakes of the inflammation which extends over the membrane generally. The appearances accompanying its inflammation have been already described. Inflammation of the peritonaeal covering of the bladder does not frequently extend to its muscular coat. The peritonaeum and the muscular coat of the bladder, are but loosely connected together, as a considerable quantity of cellular membrane is interposed between them. This loose connection is necessary, in order that the peritonaeum may be accommodated to different states of distension of the bladder, and it has also the effect of preventing inflammation from spreading readily from the peritonaeal covering of the bladder to its muscular coat. When the inflammation subsides, adhesions are frequently left behind, connecting the bladder more or less to the neighbouring parts; in a female, to the uterus, and in a male to the rectum.

Inflammation of the Inner Membrane

The inner membrane of the bladder is occasionally inflamed. When this happens, the inflammation is sometimes extended over the whole cavity, or is sometimes confined to a particular portion of it. The portion which is most frequently inflamed is that near the neck of the bladder. This may arise from two causes; the one is, that in this situation, or near it, some obstruction is frequently found to the passage of the urine, which may produce irritation, and bring on more or less of inflammation; the other is, that inflammations of the urethra occasionally extend some way within the cavity of the bladder, and even sometimes over the whole of it. It is well known that the inner membrane of the bladder, in the dead body, hardly shews vessels which are large enough to carry red blood in its natural state; but when it is inflamed it is crowded with a prodigious number of extremely fine blood vessels, and there may be sometimes seen small spots of extravasated blood. When the inflammation is in a high degree, the muscular coat of the bladder may be affected; but as this is only loosely attached to the inner membrane, the inflammation will not very readily pass from the one to the other.

Ulcers

Inflammation of the inner membrane of the bladder advances sometimes to the formation of pus, and abscesses and ulcers are occasionally produced. These, when the inflammation has been of the common sort, exhibit the ordinary appearances which have often been mentioned. They sometimes advance so far as to destroy a portion of the bladder entirely, and to form communications between it and the neighbouring parts; as with the general cavity of the abdomen, with the rectum in the male, and the vagina in the female. When the communication is formed with the general cavity of the abdomen, the urine escapes into it, producing there general peritonaeal inflammation, of which I recollect a very striking example. When the communication is formed with the vagina or the rectum, the urine will escape by these passages, producing in them more or less of irritation and inflammation.

When abscesses take place in the bladder, they are produced more frequently from local violence, than from a previous spontaneous inflammation. One of the most common causes of violence is the incision of the bladder in the operation of lithotomy. When the part has been very much irritated in the operation, or the constitution is such that it is excited to violent action by the common degree of irritation, an ulcer is formed at the lips of the wound, and spreads more or less into the cavity of the bladder.

It sometimes happens, although I believe very rarely, that the whole of the inner membrane of the bladder is destroyed by ulceration, and its muscular fibres appear as bare as if they had been nicely dissected. In the case where I recollect this process to have taken place most completely, the bladder was almost filled with a scrofulous pus. There was a curdly white matter mixed with pus, which had exactly the same appearance with that formed by the suppuration of a scrofulous absorbent gland.

Schirrhus and Cancer

From the contiguity of the bladder to parts which are very liable to schirrhus or cancer, it sometimes partakes of this disease; but I do not think that it is often singly affected by it. The disease on some occasions spreads to the bladder from the rectum, and on others from the uterus: under such circumstances the bladder becomes very thick and hard, and exhibits the ordinary cancerous structure. Communications too are generally formed either with the rectum, the uterus, or the vagina.

Fungous Excrescences

Sometimes fungous excrescences arise from the inner surface of the bladder, either in one mass, or in separate portions. Upon examination they are found to consist of a loose fibrous structure. When they are situated a little behind the neck of the bladder, which is not uncommonly the case, they must produce a considerable obstruction to the passage of the urine. A stronger action will, therefore, be required in the bladder to expel the urine. A stronger action will, therefore, be required in the bladder to expel the urine, and its muscular coat will be consequently thickened. Accordingly it is often found thickened, and it is not improbable that even where the situation of the fungus may not obstruct the passage of urine into the urethra, its presence may still irritate the bladder so as to excite it to more frequent and stronger actions than in a natural state, and the muscular coat may become thereby more or less thickened.

Polypus of the Bladder

A polypus sometimes grows from the inner surface of the bladder; but this morbid appearance occurs very rarely. I have only seen one example of it, and in this instance it filled up the greater part of the cavity of the bladder. It was very irregular in its shape, consisting of various projecting masses, and seemed pretty firm in its texture.

Elongations of the inner Membrane

I have also known the inner membrane of the bladder elongated in some parts, so as to form irregular processes. These, when cut into, were found to consist of a considerable quantity of cellular membrane, intermixed with a little fat. The process producing such an appearance was probably a slow one, and was probably also not attended with pain. If these elongations were to be situated at a distance from the neck of the bladder, they would probably not produce any inconvenience; but if situated near the neck of the bladder, they might occasion extreme difficulty in making water, and even lay the foundation of a fatal disease.

Cysts communicating with the Bladder

Cysts are sometimes found connected very intimately with the bladder, and communicating with its cavity. These in some instances have been observed to be of a large size, being perhaps half as large as the usual size of the bladder itself. There is some difficulty in explaining the manner in which they are formed. If we suppose them to be formed in the cellular membrane, upon the outside of the bladder, it is extremely difficult to explain how they should communicate with its cavity, unless by ulceration, which does not seem to take place. If we suppose them to be pouches from the bladder itself, it is still difficult, in some instances, to explain why they should be formed at all, and why they should arrive at so large a size. The latter supposition, however, seems to be the most reasonable, and I am persuaded it will apply to the greater number of cases where such cysts exist.

Muscular Coat Thickened

One of the most ordinary changes in the bladder, from its

natural structure, is the great thickening of its muscular coat. In a natural state, the muscular coat of the bladder (when it is moderately distended) consists of thin layers of muscular fibres, running in different directions. These are probably, altogether, not more than the eighth of an inch in thickness. The muscular coat of the bladder, however, is occasionally found at least half an inch thick. This arises from an additional quantity of muscle being formed in consequence or extraordinary efforts being necessary in the bladder. These efforts take place when there is any considerable difficulty in making water, as happens when the prostate gland is a good deal enlarged, when there is a stone in the bladder, or when there are strictures in the urethra. It is usual, therefore, to find this thickening of the muscular coat of the bladder when there is any of these diseases. When the bladder is thickened, the fasciculi of which its muscular coat is composed become much larger; but never, or at least very seldom, acquire the full red colour which muscles have in other parts of the body. This is a deviation from the general plan of nature with regard to the increase of muscles from exercise. When muscles are enlarged in size from exercise, they also become of a deep red colour. There is no other instance too in the body, as far as I recollect, of a muscle being so much enlarged beyond its natural size; in consequence of increased exertion, as the muscular coat of the bladder.

Between the fasciculi of the muscular fibres, little pouches are formed by the inner membrane. This arises from the pressure of the urine against the inner membrane of the bladder, which is impelled by the strong powers of the muscular coat. These pouches are often large enough to admit the end of the finger, and contain occasionally small calculi. The bladder in this state admits of very little distension, so that it is capable of containing little water; hence the inclination to make water is frequent, and frequent efforts of the muscular coat are required, which increase more and more its thickness. It is much more common to find this appearance of the bladder in the male than in the female, because in the latter there are fewer causes to produce it: since in that sex there is a want of the prostate gland altogether, and the urethra being short and wide, obstructions seldom take place in it. When the muscular coat of the bladder has been thickened, I believe that it has been sometimes mistaken for scirrhus.

The Bladder divided into two Chambers

The urinary bladder has sometimes been observed to be divided into two chambers, which communicate with each other; but this has happened very rarely. I have not had an opportunity myself of examining this singular disease, but I have received an account of such a case from Dr. Ash, which had many years ago fallen under his observation. The upper chamber of the bladder in this case was generally much distended with urine, so that a round tumour could be easily distinguished by the touch above the pubes. When a catheter was introduced into the bladder, a few ounces only of urine came away, and the tumour above the pubes remained the same as before. When the patient stood up a quart of water sometimes passed away involuntarily, the tumour very much subsided, and the complaint was for the time. After the death of the patient, the bladder was found upon examination to be divided into two chambers by a firm membranous substance, and the aperture of communication was almost obliterated.

There seem to me to be only two ways in which a division of the bladder into two chambers can happen. The one is by a morbid growth of the inner membrane, forming a ridge at some particular part, and at length by a continuation of this process, making a septum more or less complete in the bladder. I have seen the cavity of the oesophagus very much narrowed at one part by a permanent ridge being formed in its inner membrane. Something of the same kind I have also seen in a part of the small intestines. We may therefore readily admit the possibility of a similar process taking place in the inner membrane of the bladder.

Another way in which the bladder may be supposed capable of being divided into two chambers, is by a very strong contraction of its transverse muscular fibres at some particular part. This will be analogous to the hour-glass contraction of the uterus which is known occasionally to take place. When a complaint of the bladder depending upon its being divided into two chambers has been temporary, it is reasonable to suppose that it has arisen from the last cause; when it has been permanent, it is more likely to have arisen from the first.

Calculi

Calculi are not uncommonly found in the bladder, and are confined in their formation to no particular period of life. They are formed in very young children, and also in persons in middle and advanced age. This disease is not so frequently met with in the female, as in the male, which may depend on two causes; the one is, that there is not so strong a tendency to their formation in that sex; and the other cause is, that stones escape through the urethra in women, which would be detained in the bladder of men, and lay the foundation there of larger calculi.

The stones which are found in the bladder, are either originally formed in the kidneys, and pass through the ureters into the bladder, or they are first formed in the bladder itself. When the latter circumstance takes place, the earthy matter is sometimes first deposited round some extraneous body, which becomes the nucleus of the calculus, but most frequently no nucleus whatever is to be observed. The nuclei, which I have seen, have been small portions of lead (probably broken off from a leaden bougie) small nails, and little masses of hair. In short, any extraneous body which may happen to be introduced into the bladder, may become a nucleus. It is natural to think that such nuclei are more common in the calculi found in the bladder of women than of men, because their urethra is wider and shorter, so that an extraneous body can be much more easily introduced into their bladder.

The calculi of the bladder either lie loose in it, or are confined to some fixed situation from particular circumstances. When they are of a small size, they are sometimes lodged in pouches, or sacculi, formed by the protrusion of the inner membrane of the bladder between the fasciculi of its muscular fibres. A calculus also is occasionally attached to an excrescence of the bladder, so as to be kept in a fixed situation.

There is frequently one calculus only in the bladder at a time, and then it is usually of an oval form; but there are often more, and the calculi by rubbing upon each other in a narrow space acquire flat sides and angles. Calculi have sometimes a smooth uniform surface, but most frequently the surface is granulated. These granules are commonly placed very near each other over the whole surface of the calculus, giving it a certain degree of roughness. They are, however, occasionally gathered into clusters on particular parts of the surface of a calculus. These granules are sometimes of a smaller, and sometimes of a larger size, and in different calculi are more or less elevated. Some calculi have an irregular porous structure upon the surface instead of being granulated.

Calculi when divided by the saw, or broken, exhibit most commonly a laminated structure. These laminae are disposed in concentric curves, and are applied together with more or less compactness: in some calculi the laminae adhere together very slightly. They differ in their thickness in different calculi: and the laminated structure sometimes pervades uniformly the whole mass of the calculus; while at other times different portions of it are interrupted by a coarse porous texture. In some calculi no laminated structure whatever is observable, but it is entirely porous.

The colour of calculi varies considerably. They are most frequently of a brown colour, which is sometimes of a lighter, and sometimes of a darker shade. They are also sometimes of a white, and often of a yellowish colour. It is remarkable, that different portions of the same calculus are frequently of a different colour. Some laminae, for instance, are perfectly white, while the other laminae are brown. In this sort of mixture, I have most commonly found the white laminae on the outside, and the brown laminae in the middle; and I do not recollect seeing one instance of laminae of different colours, disposed in alternate strata.

The specific gravity of urinary calculi differs very considerably, as they differ a good deal in their compactness; but they are in general nearly twice the specific gravity of water.

It is only within a few years that the chemical analysis of urinary calculi has been ascertained with sufficient accuracy, and they have been found to consist of five species very different from each other.

The first species is more common than the others, and consists of a particular acid called lithic acid, mixed with some gelatinous matter, and in some instances with a very small proportion of lime. Its texture is partly laminated and partly porous. Its colour is brown, varying a good deal in the depth of its shade, and sometimes with a very slight yellowish tinge. The chemical properties of this species of urinary calculi were first ascertained by Scheele and Bergman.

The second species consists of crystals which are formed by the combination of phosphoric acid with magnesia and ammonia: these are mixed with some phosphorated lime, and generally some lithic acid. It is of a white colour, is more irregular in its shape than some of the other species, and consists partly of a laminated and partly of a porous structure. It is fusible by the blow-pipe, and therefore has commonly been called the fusible calculus.

The third species consists of the acid of sugar and acid of phosphorus united with lime; together generally with some lithic acid in the interstices. This species is knotted on its outer surface somewhat like a mulberry, and from this circumstance it has commonly been called the mulberry calculus. It is of a dark brown colour, and consists of an irregularly laminated structure. The laminae of which it is composed often vary in their colour, some of them being dark, and others of a white colour. The white laminae are commonly towards the outer part of the calculus, although its colour be dark.

The fourth species consists entirely of phosphorated lime, and has been called the bone-earth calculus. It is of a light brown colour, and its laminae slightly adhere to each other. For an accurate analysis of these three last species of urinary calculi, we are chiefly indebted to Dr. Wm. Hyde Wollaston.

The fifth species consists of carbonate of lime, mixed with a little animal matter and water, and was discovered lately by Mr. Crumpton (79).

The matter of calculus in the bladder is generally formed into one or more circumscribed masses, yet it sometimes happens that the whole bladder is filled with a substance like mortar. Of this I recollect one striking example; the earthy matter in this case could not be entirely removed from the bladder; but a great many small irregular portions still adhered to the sides of its cavity. I believe that this matter was of the same nature with a common calculus, because it exhibited the same affinities with the common acids.

79. See Thompson's System of Chemistry, Vol. 4, page 671.

Within the last three years I have met with another instance in which the matter of calculus put on the appearance and consistence of mortar, but was in small quantity. It was connected with a chronic inflammation of the inner membrane of the bladder, and processes of coagulable lymph attached to the inner membrane were encrusted with the calculous matter. This disease had continued for many years, and was combined with stricture of the urethra.

Bladder Distended

In opening dead bodies, the bladder is occasionally found to be very much distended, and to occupy the lower part of the cavity of the abdomen. This might arise from some accidental circumstance of the water being accumulated, while the muscular coat of the bladder still possessed its proper powers; or the muscular coat of the bladder may have been paralytic, and therefore not capable of expelling the water. I do not think it is possible to discriminate between these two different cases by any examination after death, but they can always be ascertained by a careful inquiry into their history.

Bladder Contracted

The bladder is also found contracted to such a degree as hardly to have any cavity. This is generally not to be considered as a disease, but simply as having arisen from a very strong action of the muscular coat of the bladder previously to death.

The anterior part of the Bladder wanting

The anterior part of the bladder is occasionally wanting, and instead of it there is a very soft vascular flesh, situated externally at the lower part of the abdomen. This soft vascular flesh is usually formed into irregular projecting masses, and in the living body is covered with a thick ropy mucus. The two ureters open somewhere upon this vascular flesh, distilling gradually the urine upon its surface, which the mucus is intended to protect against the stimulus of that fluid. When there is such a formation of the bladder, I believe that there is always a deficiency of the bone at the symphysis pubis, and also a monstrous formation of some of the organs of generation. This species of monstrosity I have described at large in the Medical and Chirurgical Transactions (80).

The Bladder and the Rectum communicating from original Malformation

Another kind of monstrous formation in the bladder occasionally happens, viz. that at its depending part there is a communication between it and the rectum, the latter being continued into the former. Of this I have seen one instance, and it has been already taken notice of when treating of the diseased and praeter-natural appearances of the intestines.

Part of the Bladder in a hernial Sack

A portion of the bladder at its fundus has been known to be lodged in a hernial sack, as well under Paupart's ligament, as at the abdominal ring; but this is very rare, and has not fallen under my own observation (81).

SYMPTOMS

In inflammation of the bladder, a pain is felt in the perinaeum, or above the pubes, accompanied with a fulness, or a swelling there. There are frequent attempts to make water, which is evacuated in small quantity and with great pain; or there is a total retention of the urine, with a strong desire to void it. The rectum is affected from its connection with the bladder and is excited to tenesmus. The stomach likewise takes a part in the disease, being affected with sickness and vomiting. In some cases there is delirium. When pus has been formed in consequence of the inflammation, it is known by being mixed with the urine which is evacuated.

80. See Med. and Chi. Trans. p. 189.
81. See Pott on Ruptures, p. 226.

When the bladder has become affected by an ulcer spreading to it from the neighbouring parts, it may be suspected by the pain and difficulty which occur in making water. When the ulcer has made a further progress, and a communication has thereby taken place between the bladder and the uterus, or between the bladder and the vagina, or between the bladder and rectum, it may be distinguished by the urine passing either through the vagina or the anus, attended with pain and irritation.

When two chambers are just beginning to be formed in the bladder, very little inconvenience is probably felt, because the communication between them at this time is very large. Under such circumstances it seems hardly possible to detect the nature of the disease in the living body; but when the disease has made a considerable progress, and the communication between the two chambers has become very narrow, it may be ascertained, or at least conjectured about with great probability, from the following circumstances. There will then be a considerable circumscribed tumour above the pubes in the situation of the bladder when distended, much less urine will be made than the natural quantity, and the tumour will not be sensibly lessened by it; or if a catheter be introduced, little urine will be evacuated, and the tumour above the pubes will still remain the same. But it will occasionally happen, by some particular attitude of the body, that the urine will pass from the upper chamber of the bladder into the lower, and from this it will be evacuated by the urethra; under such circumstances there will be a much larger quantity of urine made than usual, the tumour above the pubes will disappear, and the patient will receive immediate relief, which will continue till there is another accumulation of urine.

There are no symptoms which particularly distinguish the existence of fungous excrescences in the bladder. They produce difficulty in making water, which will be greater according as the excrescence is large, or as it is situated near the neck of the bladder. When the excrescence is very near the neck of the bladder, the disease may be ascertained by the introduction of the sound into the urethra. The extremity of the sound will come in contact with the excrescence, and will give the sensation of its pressing against a soft tumour. It may be said, that this case will with difficulty be distinguished by such an examination, from an enlargement of the prostate gland. By examining, however, into the state of the prostate gland in the usual way through the rectum, the one case may be sufficiently distinguished from the other.

The symptoms which belong to a polypus formed in the bladder, are unknown to me; but they are probably much the same with those which attend fungous excrescences in the bladder, as above described.

The symptoms which attend calculi in the bladder are well known. There is an uneasy sensation at the orifice of the urethra after making water, or after exercise. When the calculus is large, a dull pain is generally felt at the neck of the bladder. The attempts to make water are frequent, and it often passes drop by drop, or the stream is suddenly interrupted. The urine deposits a large proportion of a mucous sediment, which is produced by the mucous glands at the neck of the bladder being irritated by the calculus to an increased secretion. The urine is also occasionally tinged with blood, from some small blood vessels being ruptured by a rough part of the stone, and this is most apt to happen after some jolting motion. There is tenesmus, in consequence of the connection of the rectum with the bladder, and the sympathy which has been established between their respective functions.

When the calculous matter is soft, resembling mortar, there is great pain and difficulty in making water, which is voided frequently, and in small quantity; portions of this matter are occasionally discharged along with the urine, and generally mixed with a ropy mucus tinged with blood.

CHAPTER XV

DISEASED APPEARANCES OF THE VESICULAE SEMINALES

THE diseased appearances of the vesiculae seminales are but little known, because from their situation these bodies cannot be seen without a good deal of dissection; whereas many of the viscera come immediately into view when the cavity in which they are lodged is simply laid open: diseased appearances, however, have been occasionally observed in the vesiculae seminales.

Vesiculae Seminales inflamed

It has never occurred to me to observe the vesiculae seminales inflamed by themselves, although they are, doubtless, liable to this disease, like other parts of the body. I have seen them, however, involved in the natural consequences of inflammation with the surrounding parts. Thus I have seen the posterior surface of the bladder, the vesiculae seminales, and a portion of the rectum adhering with unusual firmness together, in the same manner as other parts of the body do after inflammation. Some few instances, however, have occurred, in which so great an inflammation had been excited in the vesiculae seminales, as to terminate in suppuration (82).

Vesiculae Seminales scrofulous

The vesiculae seminales are also affected with scrofula. I recollect to have seen one of the vesiculae seminales filled with true scrofulous matter, the distinguishing characteristic of which has been often mentioned.

---

82. See Soemmerring's Germ. Trans. p. 194.

Ducts of the Vesiculae Seminales terminating in a Cul-de-sac

The ducts of the vesiculae seminales open naturally by two distinct orifices into the cavity of the prostate gland, but they are occasionally wanting, and the vesiculae seminales terminate in a cul-de-sac. The vasa deferentia are at the same time without their natural termination, for they end in the cul-de-sac of the vesiculae seminales. This is a species of monstrosity which is very rare, but it is of great consequence, because it prevents the semen from passing into the urethra, and frustrates one of the most important functions in the animal economy. An instance of this sort of malformation is preserved in Dr. Hunter's collection.

Vesiculae Seminales very small

The vesiculae seminales differ a good deal in their size in different adult bodies, and indeed it is very common for the one to be considerably smaller than the other; but I have oftener than once seen both of them so small that they must have been very little able to fulfil the intentions for which they were formed.

One of the Vesiculae Seminales wanting

One of the vesiculae seminales is occasionally wanting altogether. Under such circumstances I believe that the extremity of the vas deferens upon that side is generally enlarged and tortuous, becoming a sort of substitute for it. This was at least the case in the instance which I have seen of this mode of formation. The extremity of the vas deferens has at all times a structure similar to that of the vesiculae seminales, and renders therefore this conjecture very probable.

Vesiculae Seminales scirrhous

The vesiculae seminales have also been observed to be scirrhous; but this is very uncommon (83).

83. See Morgagni Epist. XLVI. Art. 5.

Small stones have also been seen in the vesicular seminales, but they have not fallen under my own observation, and they are a very rare occurrence (84).

SYMPTOMS

The symptoms which attend diseases of the vesiculae seminales, have not been attempted to be discriminated by authors, and must, from circumstances, be very difficult to ascertain. It has only occurred to myself to observe some diseased changes of them in the dead body; and I have had no opportunity of tracing the symptoms which accompany these changes during life.

---

84. See Soemmerring's Germ. Trans. p. 193.

CHAPTER XVI

DISEASED APPEARANCES OF THE PROSTATE GLAND

Abscess in the Prostate Gland

THE prostate gland is not often found in a state of common inflammation. I have seen, however, an abscess in it, without any uncommon thickening and enlargement of the gland, and where the pus appeared to be of the common sort. This must be considered as being a common abscess, and must have been preceded by the ordinary sort of inflammation.

Scrofula of the Prostate Gland

The prostate gland is sometimes scrofulous. I have seen, in cutting into it, precisely the same white curdly matter, which is formed in a scrofulous absorbent gland. In squeezing it also, I have forced out from its ducts a scrofulous pus.

Scirrhus of the Prostate Gland

The most common disease of the prostate gland is a scirrhous enlargement of it. The prostate gland, it is well known, is naturally about the size of a large chestnut, but when it is attacked by scirrhus, it is often enlarged to the size of the fist. In this enlarged state, when cut into it exhibits a very firm, whitish, or brown substance, with membranous septa running through it in various directions, which are often very strongly marked. This is the common appearance of scirrhus in other parts of the body. When the prostate gland is a good deal enlarged, its cavity becomes deeper from the growth of its sides, and the posterior extremity forms a considerable projection into the cavity of the bladder, which interrupts the passage of the urine into the urethra (85). According to the degree of this projection, the urine is passed with greater or less difficulty, as well as an instrument for drawing it off. When the projection is very great, it has sometimes been found impossible to pass an instrument over the projection, and an artificial passage has been made through it accidentally, by which the urine has been evacuated. Under such circumstances the gland has been known not to be irritated by the violence used in making this new passage, and life has been prolonged for a greater length of time than it would have been otherwise. Still, however, the instrument ought to be made to pass over the projection, if possible, and we should never run the risk, by injuring the gland, of bringing on immediately fatal consequences.

Sometimes in the progress of the enlargement the prostrate gland grows irregularly, and a winding passage is formed through it, by an alteration in the shape of its cavity. This increases the difficulty to the patient of making water, and to the surgeon of introducing an instrument. When the prostate gland is enlarged, its internal surface is sometimes ulcerated, but commonly it is not (86). Fistulous communications are sometimes formed between an enlarged prostate gland and the rectum.

It is obvious too, from what has been mentioned, that in an enlarged state of the prostate gland, the difficulty of making water must be very great. This difficulty excites extraordinary and very frequent efforts in the bladder to overcome it. Its muscular coat becomes consequently much stronger and thicker, than in the natural state. A prostate gland, therefore, is never found enlarged to any considerable degree, without the bladder having undergone this change in its muscular coat. This disease is hardly ever to be found in a young person, but is not at all uncommon at an advanced period of life.

---

85. Mr. Home has lately discovered that this posterior projection is owing to the enlargment of a small separate lobule of the prostate gland, not hitherto known.

86. There seems to be little disposition to the formation of an ulcer in this state of the prostate gland. This disease may therefore be considered not improperly as in some degree different from diseases in other parts of the body, which are attended with a similar structure, but which are prone to run into ulceration.

Calculi in the Ducts of the Prostate Gland

There is another disease of the prostate gland, which occasionally takes place, although it is by no means so frequent as the former, viz. a formation of small calculi, which are lodged in its ducts. They are usually of the size of a small pea, and those which I have seen have been of a lighter or a darker brown colour. They have been found by Dr. Wm. Hyde Wollaston to consist of phosphorated lime in the state of neutralization.

Ducts of the Prostate Gland enlarged

The prostate gland is sometimes seen with its cavity very much widened, and its ducts enlarged. In the natural state of the gland, the orifices of its ducts can hardly be seen, but they sometimes are so much enlarged, as to be capable of admitting a crow quill. When the ducts are so enlarged, there is always a great obstruction to the passage of the urine through the urethra, arising most commonly from stricture there. The urine, either passing in very small quantity, or being entirely prevented from passing, is accumulated in the cavity of the prostate gland and the bladder. The effect of this accumulation is, that the cavity of the prostate gland is widened, and the ducts very much enlarged. The bladder too, from making extraordinary efforts to overcome the obstruction, has its muscular coat gradually thickened, and often to a very considerable degree. Attending, therefore, this state of the prostate gland, there is a thickened bladder, and an obstructed urethra.

The Prostate Gland preternaturally small

I have also seen the prostate gland of an extremely small size, so that it could hardly be considered as being fit for its office. It was attended with a monstrous formation of the urinary bladder and some of the organs of generation, and has been particularly described by me in the Medical and Chirurgical Transactions (87).

---

87. See page 194.

SYMPTOMS

The symptoms which attend inflammation of the prostate gland have been little taken notice of by authors. It is reasonable to think, that there will be a sense of pain more or less accute at the neck of the bladder, with much difficulty in making water, and probably tenesmus. This disease may be distinguished from a scirrhous enlargment of the prostate gland, by its quick progress, and by the pain which is felt in it.

When the prostate gland is affected with scrofula, little inconvenience is probably felt in an early state of the complaint; but if the gland should increase very considerably in its size, those symptoms must necessarily arise, which depend upon its enlargement, and which are just about to be mentioned.

When the prostate gland becomes enlarged from scirrhus, there is a difficulty in voiding the urine, and a small quantity only is discharged at a time, so that the bladder is kept always nearly full. There is sometimes a total inability to evacuate the urine. The faeces are also passed with difficulty, and when the operation is over, there is still a feeling of something more to be discharged. The straining which attends the evacuation of the urine and the faeces not unfrequently forces out some mucus, which had been secreted by this gland. A bougie or catheter is either passed into the bladder with difficulty, or on some occasions is not capable of being passed at all.

Calculi occur so rarely in the prostate gland, that their symptoms have been little taken notice of by authors. When the calculi are very small, so as to be confined entirely within the ducts of the prostate gland, it is probable that little inconvenience is produced by them. When they are large, and form a projection into the cavity of the prostate gland, there must necessarily be difficulty in voiding the urine, and there will be the same feeling when a sound or catheter is attempted to be passed into the bladder, as if an urinary calculus had got fixed or impacted in the neck of the bladder.

CHAPTER XVII

DISEASED APPEARANCES OF THE URETHRA

Abscesses

ABSCESSES are occasionally formed in the membranous part of the urethra. These may arise from an inflammation, produced by some latent cause, as abscesses are formed in any other part of the body; but they happen most frequently from an obstruction to the passage of the urine through the urethra. This obstruction is produced generally by a stricture in some part of this canal, and most frequently it is at or near the bulb of the corpus spongiosum urethrae. The urine being forced by the efforts of the bladder behind the stricture, irritates that part, producing inflammation and suppuration; the abscess breaks externally, and the urine is evacuated by this opening. While it remains in the state of an abscess, it is not at all different from any common abscess which may communicate with the bladder.

Fistulae

While the obstruction in the urethra continues, the opening made by the breaking of the abscess is not disposed to heal up, but a fistulous orifice is gradually formed. This is surrounded with parts somewhat thickened and hard, as fistulae are generally. The most common situation for these fistulous openings is behind the scrotum, because the most common situation of the stricture is at or near the bulb of the corpus spongiosum urethrae. Not uncommonly there are more than one of these openings, leading to short canals which run in different directions.

Stone in the Cavity of the membranous part of the Urethra

The cavity of the membranous part of the urethra I have seen distended into a bag large enough to contain a hen's egg. This bag was occasioned by a large stone which had lodged there. The stone had probably been driven into the cavity of the membranous part of the urethra, by the stream of urine from the bladder, but was too large to pass by the same means through the whole length of the urethra; it therefore stuck in that situation, and was gradually increased to the size which we have described, by the contact of the urine, similar to the growth of a stone in the pelvis of the ureters.

Cowper's Glands seldom observed to be diseased

I do not recollect to have seen Cowper's glands diseased, which are situated near this part of the urethra. They are doubtless liable to changes from disease, like other parts of the body; but they are small and difficult to access, so that they have very seldom become an object of examination.

Morgagni mentions one of them being converted into a ligamentous substance (88); and the excretory duct of one in another instance being obliterated (89).

Inner Membrane of the Urethra inflamed

The inner membrane of the urethra is very liable to be inflamed, particularly at its anterior extremity, and the inflammation occasionally spreads over the whole extent of the canal. This exhibits no appearance different from the inflammation of membranes lining secretory canals which open externally. The membrane is much more crowded with small blood vessels than in a natural state, and there is an increased secretion of the glands which open upon it. The inflammation is often not confined to the inner membrane of the urethra, but spreads into the substance of the corpus spongiosum, affecting both its cellular structure and its glands. Under these circumstances, the corpus spongiosum is enlarged and harder from the extravasation of the coagulable lymph into its cells, and is more vascular than in a natural state.

88. See Morgagni, Epist. XLIV. Art. 3.
89. See Morgagni, Epist. XLIV. Art. 12.

The glands, being increased in size from the inflammation, become sensible to the touch, like very small rounded tubercles.

Ulcers in the Urethra

Ulcers are also seen occasionally in laying open the urethra, but these are not frequent. This canal when inflamed has little disposition to ulcerate, as happens also to some other canals in the body, as for example the trachea.

Stricture

The most ordinary diseased appearance of the urethra is stricture. This consists in a part of the canal being narrowed, or perhaps altogether obliterated. It may take place in any part of the canal, but it is most frequent at or near the bulb of the corpus spongiosum urethrae. This stricture sometimes consists simply of an approximation of the opposite sides of the canal, so as to form a line of obstruction; at other times, the canal is narrowed for some length. The inner membrane at the stricture, sometimes exhibits the natural appearance; sometimes it is a little thickened, and occasionally its surface is abraded or ulcerated. These two last effects are generally produced by bougies; and sometimes false passages have been made into the corpus spongiosum urethrae in consequence of employing too much violence in the use of this instrument. There is often more than one stricture in the same urethra. It sometimes happens too that the stricture is more on one side of the canal than the other, so that the passage there is crooked.

Caruncle

A small fleshy excrescence sometimes grows in the urethra. This is called a caruncle, and used formerly to be considered as the most common cause of obstruction in this canal; but since dissections of dead bodies have become more frequent, it has been found in reality to be very rare.

A layer of earthy matter in the urethra

I have known one instance of a thin layer of earthy matter extending from the bladder through the whole length of the urethra.

Preternatual Orifice of the Urethra

The urethra sometimes does not open at the projecting extremity of the glans penis, but under it, where the fraenum is naturally situated; and in such cases there is no fraenum. It consists of a small rounded opening, much less than the natural termination in the glans. I have known an instance in this structure of parts, of a canal being formed besides the urethra, about two inches in length, which terminated at one extremity in a cul-de-sac, and at the other opened on the glans, where the urethra commonly does. How far this variety may be frequent I cannot pretend to determine. This deviation in the structure is not to be considered as a disease, but simply as a malformation of parts, and is not attended with any material inconvenience as far as I know.

There are some other diseased appearances of the penis, such as ulcers, phymoses, paraphymoses, &c. These are external, are very well known, and do not properly fall within my plan; I shall therefore omit them entirely.

SYMPTOMS

The symptoms, which attend the inflammation of the inner membrane of the urethra, are too well known to require being mentioned.

In stricture of the urethra there is difficulty in making water, which is greater or less according to the degree of the stricture; the stream of urine is small, sometimes forked, sometimes scattered, and sometimes the urine passes away in drops only. There is frequently also an increased secretion of mucus from the urethra, resembling a gleet. Various other symptoms may take place, in consequence of the parts in the neighbourhood of the stricture being affected; and even the constitution is sometimes much disturbed by this local irritation, exhibiting very different symptoms in different individuals.

When the urethra is obstructed by the growth of a caruncle, no symptoms are known by which it may be distinguished from a case of common stricture.

CHAPTER XVIII

DISEASED APPEARANCES OF THE TESTICLES, AND THE SPERMATIC CHORD

Hydrocele

HYDROCELE, or a collection of water in the tunica vaginalis testis, is a very common disease and is confined to no particular period of life. It is not unfrequent in very young children, and in them most commonly disappears without any chirurgical treatment. The bag in which the water is accumulated is of a pyramidical shape, and approaches more or less towards the ring of the abdominal muscle, according to the degree of the accumulation. It sometimes extends almost to the ring itself. The bag is also more or less thick in different cases: it is often scarcely thicker than the tunica vaginalis in its natural state; sometimes, when the accumulation is large, it is three or four times thicker, and is obviously laminated. In such cases too the testicle is a good deal compressed, and has sometimes been known to waste in consequence of this compression. The fluid which is accumulated is of a yellowish, a greenish, or brown colour, and resembles in its properties the serum of the blood. This disease, in persons who are advanced in life, is frequently combined with a scirrhous state of the testicle, which will be afterwards particularly described.

In almost all cases of hydrocele the water is contained in one bag, but in a few instances it has been known to be contained in several cysts. Of this I recollect a remarkable example which occurred a few years ago. This variety is probably produced by repeated partial inflammations on the inner surface of the tunica vaginalis, and occasioning adhesions, which put on the appearance of cysts.

Hydatids

Hydatids have sometimes been found in the cavity of the tunica vaginalis testis, either loose or adhering; they are, I believe, not very uncommon, but I have had no favourable opportunity of examining them accurately.

Loose Cartilages in the Tunica Vaginalis Testis

Small cartilages are sometimes found loose in the cavity of the tunica vaginalis testis, as in some of the joints in the body, more especially the knee joint. They do not however occur in the former so frequently as in the latter. They must once have been attached to some part of the inner surface of the tunica vaginalis testis, by very small processes or peduncles, and by the motion of this tunic upon the testicle they must have been separated. They afterwards continue to lie loose in the cavity of the tunica vaginalis testis, and are, I believe, attended with no inconvenience. An example of this kind has been seen by myself, and it has not unfrequently been observed by others.

Adhesions

The tunica vaginalis is frequently found adhering to the surface of the testicle. The adhesion is sometimes extended over the whole surface, but frequently consists only of scattered processes of membrane. The adhesions are sometimes fine, but sometimes they have considerable thickness, and connect the tunica vaginalis to the body of the testicle more or less closely in different cases. They are produced by some previous inflammation in the tunica vaginalis testis, as adhesions are formed after inflammation in the cavity of the chest, or the belly.

Testicle inflamed

The substance of the testicle itself is very frequently inflamed, but this disease is commonly removed by art, and hardly ever becomes an object of examination after death. It exhibits, however, precisely the same appearances as the inflammation of the substance of other parts, and therefore does not require to be particularly described. When the testicle is inflamed, the vas deferens sometimes partakes of the inflammation, its coats becoming considerably thickened, and in some instances the veins of the spermatic chord becoming varicose (90). After the inflammation of the testicle has subsided, it is not unusual for a hardness and fulness of the epidydimis to remain for a considerable length of time, or even through life. This depends on the matter which had been extravasated during the inflammation not being afterwards entirely absorbed.

Abscesses of the Testicle

Abscesses too are occasionally formed in the testicles from the progress of common inflammation, and are attended with the same circumstances as abscesses in other parts.

Testicle scrofulous

The testicle is sometimes completely changed from its natural structure, and converted into a truly scrofulous mass. Upon such occasions it is generally enlarged, and when cut into shews a white, or yellowish-white, curdly substance, which is sometimes more or less mixed with pus.

Testicle enlarged and pulpy

The testicle is sometimes much enlarged, and converted into an uniform, pulpy matter, in which its natural structure is entirely lost. This sort of change has been sometimes mistaken for scirrhus, but it is very different from what is called scirrhus in other parts of the body, and what is also found in the testicle itself.

Scirrhus and Cancer of the Testicle

The testicle is also found much enlarged, and changed into a

90. See Mr. Hunter on the Venereal Disease, p. 54.

hard mass, which is generally more or less intersected by membrane. In this there is no vestige of the natural structure, but cells are frequently observable in it containing a sanious fluid, and sometimes there is a mixture of cartilage. This state of the testicle I consider as the true scirrhus, and, according to the progress of the disease, the epidydimis and the spermatic chord are more or less, or not at all, affected. This disease not unfrequently advances to form a foul deep ulcer with thickened edges, or throws out a fungus, and then it is called the true cancer of the testicle.

Testicle cartilaginous

The testicle I have seen much enlarged, and changed into a mass of cartilage. There was also, in the case to which I allude, an ulcer near the centre of the cartilage, and in some places an imperfect appearance of cysts or cells. The cartilage did not seem different in any essential property from common cartilage, but was a little softer. This I consider as depending upon the same general diseased process with the scirrhus just described, for sometimes both structures are blended together in the same testicle.

Testicle bony

The testicle is sometimes converted into bone. A few instances only of this disease have fallen under my observation, and in them the bony process had not extended over the whole substance of the testicle, but had affected it partially.

A Cyst adhering to a Testicle containing a Vena Medinensis

I have seen a testicle with a small firm cyst adhering to it, which contained a worm of that sort called vena medinensis. This is a worm of considerable length, with a smooth surface, and an uniform appearance; at the posterior extremity it terminates in a slender hood-like process, and at the anterior, there is a rounded opening or mouth. This testicle had probably belonged to a man who had visited some of those climates in which the vena medinensis is found, and who had brought it over with him to this country.

The Epidydimis ending in a Cul-de-sac

The testicles have sometimes this sort of mal-formation, that the epidydimis does not terminate in a vas deferens, but in a cul-de-sac. In these cases it is evident that the semen cannot be evacuated by the urethra, and that the person must therefore be incapable of procreation. In Dr. Hunter's collection, a preparation of this sort is preserved; and Mr. Hunter has given a representation of it in his Animal Economy (91).

Stricture of the Vas Deferens

I have also seen a portion of the canal of the vas deferens obliterated by stricture. This had not been an original fault, but was the effect of a diseased process, similar probably to that which produces stricture in the urethra, and must have prevented the semen of one of the testicles from reaching the cavity of the prostate gland.

Testicles very small, and wasted

The testicles are sometimes exceedingly small in their size. I have known one case, in a person of middle age, where each of them was not larger than the extremity of the finger of an adult. This, as appeared from its history, arose from a fault in the original formation, and was attended with a total want of the natural propensities. It is much more common for a testicle to waste either spontaneously, or in consequence of a previous inflammation or compression, so as gradually to disappear entirely (92). When this takes place in one testicle only, the natural powers are preserved; but when it takes place in both, they must be altogether lost.

Sometimes one testicle, and sometimes both, remain in the cavity of the abdomen through life, so that a person appears to have only one testicle, or to be without them altogether. The testicle or testicles, I believe, are in these cases of a small size; and

91. See page 47, plate V.
92. See Hunter on the Venereal Disease, p. 209.

Mr. Hunter suspects that they are by no means so perfect as when they descend into the scrotum (93).

DISEASED APPEARANCES OF THE SPERMATIC CHORD

Spermatic Chord Scirrhous

The spermatic chord is also liable to diseased alterations of structure: one of the most common is that of its becoming scirrhous. This I believe to be very rarely, if at all, an original disease of the chord, but always, or almost always, spreads to it from the testicle. In the early state of a scirrhous testicle the spermatic chord is perfectly sound; but when the disease has existed for a considerable time, and does not remain stationary, the chord becomes at length affected. Under such circumstances it is changed into a hard mass, exhibiting the same appearance of structure as the testicle itself. During the last stage the disease advances to the loins, so as to affect the absorbent glands there.

Veins of the Spermatic Chord varicose

The disease of the spermatic chord which is not uncommon, is an enlargement of its veins. The veins of the spermatic chord are numerous, and support a very long column of blood. This last circumstance, added to some impediments which occasionally take place to the return of the blood, renders the veins frequently enlarged. This enlargement varies very much in different cases, arising from the degree and the continuance of the impediment. When the enlargement of the veins is very considerable, they also become varicose, and the spermatic chord is changed into a bulky mass, soft to the feeling, and capable of being readily diminished upon pressure. In this state of the spermatic chord, the testicle is sometimes wasted.

Water accumulated in the cellular Membrane of the Spermatic chord

Water has sometimes been known to be accumulated in the cells

93. See Mr. Hunter's Observations on certain parts of the Animal Economy, p. 18.

of the cellular membrane, which envelopes the vessels of the spermatic chord. The cellular membrane of this part of the body is in considerable quantity, and when water is accumulated in its cells, a large swelling is formed in the situation of the spermatic chord, which is readily diminished upon pressure. When pressure is used, the swelling is diminished, not only by a part of the water being forced into the cells of the chord within the abdominal ring, but also by its being forced into the cellular membrane under the skin of the lower part of the belly. Many pints have been known to be accumulated in these cells. It has never occurred to myself to see this disease, and therefore I have had no opportunity of examining the nature of the fluid; but I presume it is of the same sort with what is usually found in anasarca.

A Sack containing water formed in the Spermatic chord

A sack has also been known to be formed in the spermatic chord, consisting of a firm, white membrane, and containing a fluid which most probably is of a serous nature. Both of these cases have been particularly described by Mr. Pott, in his treatise upon Hydrocele (94).

SYMPTOMS

The existence of hydrocele in the living body, may be determined by the shape of the tumour, which is in some degree pyramidal, by the resistance which it gives upon pressure, by the want of pain in it, and by the health being not affected by it. Where the tunica vaginalis is thin, and the swelling is placed between the eye and a lighted candle, it will appear transparent. Where the tunica vaginalis, however, is thick, the transparency will be lost, and the tumour to the feeling will be harder, and less compressible. But still it will not have the same degree of hardness as a scirrhous testicle, and will want some other characteristic marks which belong to the latter disease.

The formation of hydatids in the tunica vaginalis testis is

94. For the first case, see Pott on Hydrocele, p. 39. For the second, see Pott on Hydrocele, p. 57.

attended with symptoms which correspond very much with those of hydrocele; and this case can only be distinctly known by laying open the sack.

An inflamed testicle may be distinguished from a scirrhous one in the living body, by a slight attention to the appearances, and to the history of the case. The progress of the disease, in an inflamed testicle, is commonly rapid, and the skin of the scrotum immediately covering it has usually a blush of inflammation; but in a scirrhous testicle, the progress of the disease is slow, and the skin of the scrotum retains its natural colour, unless it be really affected by the disease. The surface of the tumour in an inflamed testicle is uniform and smooth, but in a scirrhous testicle is often irregular.

When a testicle is scrofulous or pulpy, it may be distinguished from a scirrhous testicle by its greater softness, by the little pain which is felt in it, and by the health being usually pretty good, even when the disease has been of long standing.

A scirrhous testicle may be ascertained in the living body, by its great hardness, and by the pain that is often felt in it, which darts along the spermatic chord to the loins. Its progress is commonly slow, the spermatic chord becomes ultimately diseased, and the general health at length much impaired. When it throws out a fungus, or forms an ill-conditioned ulcer, these become additional external marks of the nature of the disease.

The encysted tumour of the spermatic chord, containing water, resembles, in some appearances, hydrocele. It may, however, be distinguished from it by the testicle being felt separate and entire under the tumour, which in hydrocele is never the case.

CHAPTER XIX

DISEASED APPEARANCES IN THE FEMALE ORGANS

Inflammation of the Uterus

WHEN the uterus becomes inflamed, it takes place almost always under the same circumstances, viz. very soon after parturition. The inflammation is sometimes confined to the uterus itself, or its appendages, but the peritonaeum in the neighbourhood is most commonly affected, and frequently over its whole extent. The uterus, when inflamed, exhibits the same appearance as the inflammation of the substance of other parts, and these are principally observable in its body or fundus. The inflammation is frequently found to creep along the appendages of the uterus, especially the Fallopian tubes and ovaria. It often advances to suppuration, and the pus is generally found in the large veins of the womb (95). When the peritonaeum is also affected by inflammation, it exhibits the same appearances which we formerly described particularly when treating of the inflammation of this membrane; but the extravasated fluid, and the coagulable lymph, are not uncommonly in very large proportion to the degree of the inflammation (96).

Malignant Ulcer of the Uterus

It is not unusual for an ulcer to be formed in the uterus, of a very malignant nature. This is most apt to happen in women at the middle period of life, or a more advanced age; but it sometimes happens in women who may still be said to be young. The ulcer

---

95. Dr. Clarke's Essays, p. 69 and 70.

96. Dr. Clarke, who has examined a great many women that have died after parturition with inflammation of the peritonaeum, has observed this particularly. See Dr. Clarke's Essays, p. 136.

generally begins in the cervix uteri, and the uterus is at the same time somewhat harder and larger than in the natural state. It does not, however, grow to any considerable size. The ulcer spreads from the cervix to the fundus uteri, and it is not unusual to see the greater part of the fundus destroyed by it, the rest being changed into a tattered ulcerated mass. The ulceration is not always confined in its boundaries to the uterus, but sometimes spreads into the neighbouring parts, as the vagina, the bladder, and the rectum, making communications between them, and producing dreadful havock. This disease of the uterus is generally considered as cancer, but it differs in some of its appearances from what is acknowledged to be the true cancer in other parts of the body (97).

Scirrhous Enlargement of the Uterus

It sometimes happens, although not very often, that the uterus enlarges in its size, and becomes much harder than in its natural state. This change corresponds very much to that of scirrhus in other parts of the body, and commonly extends over the whole of the uterus. It is difficult to say to what size the uterus may at length arrive, in the progress of this disease, but I have seen it, in one case, as large as the gravid uterus at the sixth month. If a transverse section be made of the uterus in this state, it is found to consist of a hard substance, intersected by pretty thick membranes. Ulceration is sometimes discovered upon its inner surface, but I believe it is commonly wanting. Tubercles are occasionally formed in this state of the uterus, being, as it were, imbedded in its substance, and they have a structure very much resembling that of the uterus itself.

Tubercles of the Uterus

Hard tubercles often grow from the uterus, which are either

97. This diseased change I formerly confounded with the scirrhous enlargement of the uterus, considering them as varieties of the same disease, and therefore blending their description together; but in consequence of the accurate observations of Dr. Adams, in his Essays upon Morbid Poisons, I have thought it proper to separate them.

imbedded in its substance, or arise from its outer surface. They vary a good deal in their size, viz. from that of a hazel nut to more than the size of the fist. They are irregular in their shape, but are commonly rounded, and are often in some degree knotted. These, when cut into, exhibit a hard whitish substance, intersected by membranous septa, which are commonly very thick and strong. They seem to have little disposition to ulceration, for they are very rarely found affected by this process. The uterus in this state of disease, is generally of the natural size, and possesses the healthy structure, but occasionally it is much enlarged.

A mass of the same kind is sometimes found in the cavity of the uterus, and often grows to a very large size. I have seen it a good deal larger than a child's head at birth. This mass when cut into, exhibits precisely the same appearance as these we have so lately described. It is remarkable, that such masses within the cavity of the uterus commonly do not adhere in any part closely to it, but are connected with it loosely, by the intervention of cellular membrane, and small blood vessels, so that they can be very easily peeled off, without injuring the structure of the uterus. The uterus itself is more or less enlarged according to the bulk of the mass it contains, but it appears to be perfectly healthy in its structure.

Polypus

Polypus forms a very common disease of the uterus, and may take place almost at any period of life; it is more frequent, however, at the middle or advanced age, and rarely happens in persons who are young. By a polypus is meant a diseased mass, which adheres to some part of the cavity of the uterus, by a sort of neck or narrower portion. It is of different kinds: the most common kind is hard, and consists of a substance, divided by thick membranous septa. When cut into, it shews precisely the same structure as the tubercle of the uterus just described; so that a person looking upon a section of the one and the other out of the body, could not at all distinguish between them. This sort of polypus varies very much in its size, some being not larger than a walnut, and others being larger than a child's head. It adheres by a narrower portion or neck, which varies a great deal in its size, and in its proportion to the body of the polypus. The largest polypus I ever saw was suspended by a neck hardly thicker than the thumb; and I have seen a polypus, less than the fist, adhering by a neck fully as thick as the wrist.

The place of adhesion also differs considerably. It is most commonly at the fundus uteri, but it may take place in any other part; and I have seen a small polypus adhering just on the inner part of the lip of the os uteri. When a polypus is of any considerable size, there is generally one only; but I have occasionally seen on the inside of the uterus, two or three small polypi, and in some instances, several polypi have been known to grow from the uterus in succession.

Another sort of polypus takes place in the uterus, which consists of an irregular, bloody substance, with a number of tattered processes hanging from it. This when cut into exhibits two different appearances of structure: the one appearance is that of a spongy mass, consisting of laminae, with small interstitial cavities between them; the other is that of a very loose texture, consisting of large irregular cavities. It is very obvious that, in proportion as a polypus grows, the cavity of the uterus must be enlarged, and the same change must take place in the vagina, when a polypus protrudes from the uterus into this canal.

The Inversion of the Uterus

The inversion of the uterus occasionally takes place, and principally from two causes, viz. from the weight of a polypus, or from violent pulling in attempts to remove the placenta. When the inversion is incomplete, the fundus uteri forms a tumour within its cavity; there is at the same time an appearance of fissure upon the outside of the uterus, where the fundus usually is; and the Fallopian tubes, the round ligaments, and the ligaments of the ovaria, are drawn inwards at both edges of the fissure. The uterus, particularly after labour, is sometimes inverted entirely, the inner surface being exposed, and the fundus uteri forming a large tumour within the vagina, and in some cases even on the outside of the labia.

Prolapsus Uteri

The uterus sometimes leaves its natural situation and falls downwards, so as either to get to the external parts, or out of the body entirely. This is most apt to happen when women have a large pelvis, and where the soft parts have been very much relaxed by repeated and severe labours. This disease is called prolapsus uteri, and will be explained more particularly when we come to treat of the diseases of the vagina. It is much more frequent than the other disease called the inversio uteri.

Stricture in the cavity of the Uterus

A stricture is sometimes formed within the cavity of the uterus, so that its cavity at one part is obliterated entirely. This I believe almost always to take place at one part, viz. where the cavity of the fundus uteri terminates, and that of the cervix begins, for in this place the cavity of the uterus is narrowest. As the sides of the cavity round this place lie very near each other, and form naturally a small aperture, it is probable that some slight inflammation may unite the parts together, and shut up the aperture; or the parts may gradually approach each other without this cause, as in strictures of the urethra.

The Os Uteri contracted, and closed up

The os uteri has been found to be so contracted, as to have its passage in a great measure obliterated (98); and it has even been known to be closed up, by the growth of an adventitious membrane (99).

Uterus bony

The substance of the uterus is sometimes more or less converted into bone. This arises from a particular morbid action of its blood vessels, by which they secrete from the blood bony matter, and it is a very rare disease.

98. Vid. Morgagni, Epist. LXVII. Art. 11.
99. Vid. Morgagni, Epist. XLVI. Art. 17.

The Uterus changed into an earthy Substance

The uterus has also been known to be converted into an earthy substance (100). It is probably of the same kind with the earth of bones; and this disease probably differs only from the former, in their being a less proportion of animal gluten, to combine the earthy particles together.

A bony mass in the Cavity of the Uterus

In the cavity of the uterus a bony mass is sometimes found. When this is the case, I suspect that the hard fleshy tubercle within the cavity of the uterus, such as we have lately described, has been converted into bone. This at least had taken place in the only instance which I have known of it, (for a great part of the tubercle still remained unchanged) and I think it very probable, that such a change most frequently happens where these bony tumours are found.

Stones in the Cavity of the Uterus

Stones (101) have sometimes been found in the cavity of the uterus. These are described by authors as varying in their appearance, some being of a dark, and others of a light colour. About their nature they are silent, and I can say nothing of it from my own knowledge, as it has never occurred to me to see an instance of this disease. Such concretions are probably formed from matter thrown out by the small arteries which open upon the internal surface of the uterus, and are in some degree analogous to the concretions which are formed in some glands of the body.

Dead Foetus in the Uterus converted into an earthy Mass

It has also been known to happen, that a dead foetus has remained for a long time in the cavity of the uterus, and has there been gradually changed into an earthy mass preserving the shape of the child (102).

100. Vid. Lieutaud, Tom. I. p. 323.
101. Vid. Lieutaud, Tom. I. p. 339.
102. See Cheselden's Anatomy of the Bones, plate LVI.

Water in the Cavity of the Uterus

Water has sometimes been known to be accumulated in the cavity of the uterus in very large quantity (103). In some cases fifty, sixty, or even a hundred pints have been said to be accumulated. This water is sometimes bloody in its appearance, and sometimes of a yellowish colour. Of its nature I cannot speak particularly, as I have never seen an instance of this disease. I think it probable, however, that the water accumulated in the cavity of the uterus, resembles in its properties the serum; and that it is poured out by the small curling arteries of the uterus. In cases where water is really accumulated in the cavity of the uterus, one must suppose a stricture of the cervix, otherwise the water would escape gradually into the vagina as it is formed. I am disposed to believe, however, that where water has been said to be accumulated in the cavity of the uterus, it has frequently been really in one or more large hydatids formed in that cavity (104).

Hydatids in the Uterus

Large masses of hydatids (105) have also been found in the cavity of the uterus. Whether these be commonly of the same kind with what occasionally grow in the placenta, or like those in the other parts of the body, I cannot determine, as it has not occurred to me to see an example of this disease. The hydatids of the placenta are a good deal different from those of the liver, kidneys, and some other parts of the body. They consist of vesicles of a round or oval shape, with a narrow stalk to each, by which they adhere on the outside of one another. Some of these hydatids are as large as a walnut, and others as small as a pin's head. A large hydatid has generally a number of small hydatids adhering to it by narrow processes. Of their real nature nothing is known, but they are probably animals of a very simple structure. In the same quadruped sometimes different species of hydatids will occur, and

103. Vid. Lieutaud, Tom. I. p. 319, p. 333.

104. Dr. Denman has had an opportunity of observing a case, where water was accumulated in one large hydatid of the uterus.

105. Vid. Lieutaud, Tom. I. p. 335.

therefore the same thing may take place in the human subject. I believe that the hydatids said to be found in the uterus, have not uncommonly been only hydatids of the placenta, which has been retained there.

Rupture of the Uterus

These are the various diseased appearances which are well ascertained to take place in the uterus. I have to add, that the womb is not unfrequently ruptured, which is rather to be considered as an accident than a disease. This, perhaps, never takes place but in the pregnant uterus, and at the time of delivery. It may arise either from too violent an action of the muscular fibres of the uterus upon the child, or upon the hand of an accoucheur, who may for some reason or other have introduced it into its cavity. The ruptures which I have seen have been commonly in the side of the womb, and of considerable extent. The peritonaeum covering the womb sometimes remains whole, and there is a large mass of black coagulated blood lying between it and the uterus, where the rupture has taken place. This black appearance is occasionally mistaken for mortification.

Two Uteri

It has sometimes happened, although very rarely, that two uteri have been formed in the same person instead of one. In this case there is but one ovarium and one Fallopian tube to each. The vagina is at the same time divided by a septum into two canals, each of which conducts to its proper uterus. In the case which is described in the Philosophical Transactions (106), a communication was formed at one part through the septum; but how far this generally takes place in such a kind of monstrosity I cannot determine.

Natural Varieties in the Uterus

The uterus varies a good deal in its size in different persons, in

106. See Philosoph. Trans. Vol. LXIV. p. 474.

some being fully twice as large as it is in others. It differs also somewhat in the thickness of its substance. There is some difference too in its situation, being often placed nearer one side of the pelvis than the other. All of these are to be considered as varieties in the natural formation, and not as disease.

SYMPTOMS

In inflammation of the uterus, there is a sense of pain and tension in the hypogastric region, and the pain is increased upon pressure there, or upon touching the os uteri. The stomach is affected with vomiting, and the bowels are sometimes as costive, and sometimes disposed to looseness. The whole constitution is roused into action, exhibiting those symptoms which have been called fever, and the pulse has commonly a great degree of frequency. When the peritonaeum is inflamed over the general surface of the abdomen, or to a considerable extent, there is a general swelling of that cavity, with pain and extreme tenderness upon pressure, and the feverish symptoms are increased.

In the malignant ulcer of the uterus there is a sense of pain in the hypogastric region, which is often very violent. At the same time there is commonly felt a dull pain round the hips and down the thighs. Mucus, pus, and blood are frequently discharged by the vagina, and the quantity of blood is sometimes very large. The pulse at the beginning of this dreadful disease is natural and the general health is but little impaired, but when it is far advanced the pulse becomes quick, the countenance sallow, and the body emaciated.

If in the progress of the disease a communication should be formed between the vagina and the urinary bladder, the urine will then pass off by the vagina. Some of the glands of the groin in advanced stages of the disease often become hard and enlarged in their size.

In the scirrhous enlargement of the uterus, there are few symptoms to characterise it till the disease has made considerable progress. There is pain in the hypogastric region and round the hips, which is more or less acute in different cases; but this is common to it with several other diseases. When the disease, however, is a good deal advanced, it may be ascertained by an examination by the vagina. The os tincae will then feel enlarged and hard, and there will be an unusual sense of weight against the finger from the increased size of the uterus. A tumour may at the same time be distinctly felt above the pubes. This disease is commonly attended with mucous discharges from the vagina, and profuse discharges of blood at the monthly periods. The pulse is generally natural, and the health not much impaired.

When tubercles are formed in the uterus, and the uterus remains of its natural size, there are, I believe, no symptoms which particularly characterize this disease. But when the uterus is at the same time much enlarged, the symptoms are the same with those which belong to the common state of a scirrhous uterus, as above described.

The symptoms which attend a polypus of the uterus, are mucous and occasional bloody discharges by the vagina, with frequent pains round the hips. When it has made considerable progress in its growth, it may be ascertained by an examination by the vagina. Even without this examination, it may be distinguished from an ulcer of the uterus, by attention to the history of its progress, and by the general health being much less affected in this case than when an ulcer has been formed. The glands of the groin are, I believe, never affected from a polypus, but are often tainted by absorption, in advanced stages of the ulcerated uterus.

When there is a part of the fundus uteri inverted, forming a tumour in the cavity of the uterus, there are no symptoms by which it can be sufficiently distinguished in the living body. It is attended with a profuse haemorrhage, and if the patient should survive, the menstrual flux is in very large quantity, together with very copious mucous discharges in the intermediate times. When the inversion is complete, it can be ascertained by an examination of the tumour, but is not distinguished by any peculiar symptoms. The attempts which have been made to return the uterus to its natural situation, have almost always been unsuccessful.

Prolapsus uteri can always be ascertained by an examination, and the exact circumstances attending this case cannot be ascertained without it.

There are no symptoms by which dropsy of the uterus can be

distinguished from some other conditions of this organ, and therefore it is only known in consequence of the evacuation of the water.

There will of course be more or less enlargement of the uterus, and fulness of the hypogastric region, in proportion to the accumulation of the water, and this will subside when the water is evacuated.

The existence of hydatids in the uterus is not distinguished by any characteristic symptoms, and is only known in consequence of their expulsion, by the contractile power of this viscus. This generally takes place, and is attended with pains resembling very much the pains of labour.

A rupture of the uterus can only be fully ascertained by an examination. It is attended with pain, with a sense of something having given way in the belly, and with almost an immediate vomiting of a chocolate-coloured matter. The uterus gives up its natural efforts for the expulsion of the child, so that the labour pains cease; the child is retracted, and generally escapes, either wholly or in part, into the cavity of the abdomen.

CHAPTER XX

DISEASED APPEARANCES OF THE OVARIA

Inflammation of the Peritonaeal covering of the Ovaria

THE portion of the peritonaeum which covers the ovaria I believe is seldom inflamed, unless where the inflammation has spread to it from the uterus, or where it has attacked this membrane generally. It is not unusual, however, for it to be inflamed under both of these circumstances; and it shews the same appearances as the inflammation of the peritonaeum covering any other part. Adhesions too are frequently found, joining the ovaria to the neighbouring parts, which had been the consequence of such an inflammation.

Inflammation of the substance of the Ovaria

Where the uterus has been inflamed to a considerable degree, as after parturition, the substance of the ovaria has also been occasionally attacked by the inflammation spread to it. The ovaria are then enlarged, are harder than in a natural state, and are highly vascular; very commonly pus is found to have been formed.

Scirrhus of the Ovaria

Scirrhus is a disease which sometimes attacks the ovaria, although seldom in comparison of its attacking the uterus. Under such circumstances the ovaria become enlarged, and are converted into a whitish hard mass, which is more or less intersected with membranous septa. These scirrhous masses have sometimes a disposition to be converted into bone; and in this way most frequently, I believe, the ovaria become bony. The bony substance into which they are converted has sometimes a greater admixture of earth than the natural bones of the body.

Ovaria enlarged and changed into a pulpy Substance

The ovaria are sometimes very much enlarged, and converted into pulpy matter of a smooth uniform texture. Cells are often formed in a part of this substance, which contain a fluid.

Ovaria Scrofulous

The ovaria are sometimes changed into a true scrofulous matter, intermixed with cells.

Dropsy of the Ovaria

The most common disease of the ovaria is dropsy. The whole substance of an ovarium is sometimes destroyed, and it is converted into a capsule containing a fluid. The capsule is frequently of a large size: it consists of a white firm membrane, and contains an aqueous fluid, capable of being partly coagulated.

When the substance of the ovaria is destroyed, and they become dropsical, it is very common for them to be converted into a number of cells, which communicate with each other by considerable openings, and to be prodigiously enlarged. An ovarium in this case may be so increased in size as to occupy almost the whole cavity of the abdomen. The ovaria are also sometimes converted into a congeries of cysts, which have no communication with each other. These vary a good deal in their size, some being not larger than a hazel nut, and others as large as an orange. Their coats are sometimes thin, sometimes of considerable thickness, and consist of a compact, white, laminated membrane. They contain either a serous fluid, with which I have seen some slimy matter mixed, or a thick ropy fluid, or a kind of jelly. This jelly is sometimes so tough that it can be drawn out to a considerable length, and when it breaks, it passes back with a great deal of elastic force. Different cysts in the same ovarium will sometimes contain different sorts of fluid, a circumstance which one would not expect *a priori.*

These cysts, I believe, have been occasionally confounded with hydatids, to which they bear some resemblance. They are however really very different. They have much firmer and less pulpy coats than hydatids; they contain a different kind of fluid, and they are differently connected among themselves. Hydatids either lie unconnected with each other, or a large hydatid incloses a number of smaller ones; or smaller hydatids adhere to the coats of those which are larger. Cysts of the ovarium adhere to each other laterally by pretty broad surfaces; do not inclose each other; and appear to have no power analogous to generation as hydatids have, by which smaller cysts are formed, that are attached to those of a larger size. It appears not improbable, that these cysts are formed by a gradual enlargement of the small vesicles of which make a part of the natural structure of the ovaria.

The Ovaria changed into a fatty Substance with Hair and Teeth

The ovaria are sometimes converted into a fatty substance, intermixed with long hair and teeth, which is surrounded by a capsule consisting of a white strong membrane. The hairs are most of them loose in the fatty substance, but many of them also adhere on the inside of the capsule. Teeth too are formed, but are generally incomplete, the fangs being wanting. These sometimes arise immediately from the inner membrane of the capsule, and are sometimes connected with an irregular mass of bone. Such productions have been commonly considered as very imperfect ova, in consequence of impregnation; but there is good reason to believe that they can take place without any intercourse between the sexes. I have described a case, which has been published in the Philosophical Transactions, where it was hardly possible that impregnation could have happened. The girl in whom this change of the ovarium was found could not from all appearances have been more than twelve or thirteen years old; the hymen was perfect; and the uterus had not received that increase of bulk which is usual at puberty. The other marks of puberty were also wanting. From these circumstances I should judge the womb to have been incapable of the stimulus of impregnation. A tumour, consisting of teeth and hair, was preserved by the celebrated

Ruysch (107) in his collection, which he says was found in a man's stomach. If this be true (which there seems to be no reason to doubt,) it puts my conjecture beyond dispute. This production could not possibly, under such circumstances, have any connection with impregnation; and if it occurs without it in one part of the body, there can be no good reason why it may not also take place without impregnation in another part. These productions are much more frequent in the ovaria than any where else, probably because the process which forms them bears some analogy to generation, in which the ovaria are materially concerned. I must still therefore, whatever objections have been made to it, retain my former opinion. These masses in the ovaria are commonly about the size of a large orange (108).

107. Vid. Ruysch, Tom. II. Adversar. Anatomicor. Decad. tert.

108. I have very lately met with the same kind of fatty substance intermixed with hair, and the body of one tooth covered with enamel, in the ovarium of a young woman about eighteen years of age. In this case the uterus was rather less than its usual size in the adult when unimpregnated, and there was no membrana decidua whatever formed in its cavity. It appeared, therefore, to be undergoing no change similar to what happens when there is an ovum growing in the ovarium or the Fallopian tube. The human too was perfect, the edge of the membrane being quite sound and natural, and the aperture in it being remarkably small. These circumstances do not amount to demonstrative evidence, but still must be considered as a very strong confirmation of the truth of the opinion above stated.

I have been informed by Mr. Colman, that a dead gelding was some time ago examined, in which a cyst was found a little under the right kidney, containing a fatty matter, hair, and some teeth. This fully establishes the truth of the opinion above stated.

The particulars discovered by dissection are very curious, and are so clearly stated by Mr. Colman, that I shall take the liberty of subjoining the account of them in his own words:

"A bay gelding, seven years old, belonging to the Royal Horse Artillery at Woolwich, was attacked with a contagious and incurable disease, (viz glanders) in consequence of which I recommended that the horse should be destroyed. After the morbid parts concerned in this disease had been examined, Mr. Percivall, Veterinary Surgeon to the most honourable Board of Ordnance, (whose attention to anatomy and his profession in general deserves the highest encomiums) accidentally opened the cavity of the abdomen, and discovered a tumour about the size of a horse's testicle, of an oblong form, a little below the right kidney, and loosely attached, by a long slender neck, to the peritonaeum. Mr. Percivall removed this tumour without supposing that the contents were peculiar, but as the inner parts felt as if they were of a bony nature, a longitudinal section was made with a saw completely through its substance. It now appeared the outer cyst of the tumour contained two small molar horse-teeth, and one incisor tooth, with a portion of bone attached to this tooth resembling the jaw. The remainder of the tumour was composed of about two thirds of fat, and one third of hair of a black colour contained in a separate cyst. The molar teeth, which were fortunately

A Foetus in the Ovarium

A foetus is sometimes found in the ovarium – this seldom arrives at the full size, but its formation as far as it goes is commonly perfect. When this happens, all vestige of the ovarium is lost, and instead of it there is a bag of some firmness containing the foetus; to this bag, upon the inside, is attached a placenta, and a part of the chorion. The bag can be ascertained to be the ovarium by tracing upon it the Fallopian tube and the spermatic vessels, from their origin to their termination. The uterus in such cases is considerably larger than when unimpregnated, and in its cavity there is formed the membrana decidua. This shews that the uterus takes on the same changes, although imperfectly, which it does in the ordinary circumstances of pregnancy. The spermatic vessels are also enlarged, in order to supply a sufficient quantity of blood to the ovum which is growing in the ovarium.

Shrinking of the Ovaria

The ovaria commonly shrink towards old age, and are changed in their structure. They are diminished to half their natural size, are somewhat tuberculated on their surface and are hard. When cut into, the vesicles, which make a part of their natural structure, are found to be filled with a white solid matter.

One Ovarium or both wanting

An ovarium on one side has been known to be wanting; but this

---

divided by the saw longitudinally near the centre, had the same arrangement of enamel and bony matter as natural horse's teeth. Two very small blood vessels were observed going from the neck of the tumour into its substance, but they were not attended to, till the section had been made. As the history of the animal from its birth could not be procured, it cannot be ascertained whether both testicles had previously been removed. It is possible that one testicle might have remained in the abdomen, and the form, situation, and size of the tumour, rather favour this supposition.

But whether blood vessels were formed from the neighbouring parts to produce this peculiar organization, or whether the teeth and hair were produced by the spermatic vessels, the process is equally curious and inexplicable, This phenomenon, however, fully establishes the opinion of Dr. Baillie, that when teeth and hair and fat are found in the ovaria, impregnation is not necessary to their formation, and therefore it is highly probable, that in no instance it has been the cause of these extraordinary productions in the ovaria."

is extremely rare. An example of this kind is preserved in Dr. Hunter's collection. Some instances have been recorded, in which no vestige of an ovarium could be observed on either side.

SYMPTOMS

As the ovaria are very seldom inflamed, unless when inflammation has at the same time attacked the uterus; it is not known whether there be any particular symptoms which characterize inflammation of the ovaria. Inflammation of the ovaria cannot at present be distinguished, by its symptoms from inflammation of the uterus.

A scirrhous state of the ovaria, is with difficulty determined in the living body. When a scirrhous ovarium has increased to a large size, and lies upon the side of the pelvis, and the person is at the same time of a spare habit, it may in some measure be ascertained by an accurate examination of the tumour through the parietes of the abdomen. The tumour will feel much harder than where an ovarium is enlarged by dropsy, or filled with cysts. When the ovarium is not capable of being accurately examined, the opinion about the existence of this disease must rest much more upon probable evidence than upon any clear proof.

Dropsy of the ovarium cannot be ascertained in a very early stage of this disease. But when it has made considerable progress, so as to have formed a swelling at the lower part of the belly, it may commonly be ascertained by an accurate examination, and attention to the history of its growth. The tumour is generally on one side of the abdomen more than the other, according as the right or left ovarium is affected. There is often an inequality in the surface of the swelling, and an obscure kind of fluctuation is felt upon striking with the hand the parietes of the abdomen, which cover the swelling. The health is commonly very little affected by this disease, and it is slow in its progress, so that life will often be continued with tolerable comfort under it for many years. The quantity of the urine is often but little diminished below what is usual in health, and the absorbents of the ovarium are hardly capable of being excited to a vigorous action by medicine. There have been few instances, therefore, of a dropsy of the ovarium being cured.

CHAPTER XXI

DISEASED APPEARANCES OF THE FALLOPIAN TUBE

Inflammation of the Fallopian Tubes

WHEN the uterus is inflamed to a considerable degree, the inflammation often spreads along the Fallopian tubes: they become, in this case, highly vascular, and, when cut open, sometimes contain blood in their cavities. The inflammation may even advance to suppuration, when their cavities will be found loaded with pus.

Adhesions

When the peritonaeum generally, or some part of it, in the neighbourhood of the Fallopian tubes, is inflamed, the external covering of these tubes, which is a continuation of the peritonaeum, also partakes of the inflammation. This, when it subsides, generally terminates in adhesions of the Fallopian tubes to the contiguous parts. It is not unusual to find the fimbriated extremity of the Fallopian tubes adhering to the ovaria; or when the previous inflammation has been considerable, to find the fimbriated appearance entirely lost, and the body of the Fallopian tube apparently terminating on the surface of the ovarium. Under such circumstances there is no aperture towards this end of the Fallopian tubes and it has lost its power of conveying the ovum from the ovarium to the uterus.

The very small aperture by which the Fallopian tube communicates with the cavity of the uterus, is sometimes obliterated, but not so often as the aperture of that extremity next to the ovarium.

Dropsy of the Fallopian Tubes

When the Fallopian tube has its apertures closed at both

extremities, it is sometimes dilated into a considerable tortuous cavity. This when laid open appears occasionally subdivided by small partial septa, and contains an aqueous fluid, which is capable of being partly coagulated. This fluid is undoubtedly supplied by the secretion of the small arteries belonging to the inner membrane of the Fallopian tube, which is naturally very vascular. It may be called dropsy of the Fallopian tube.

The Fallopian tubes terminating in a Cul-de-sac

The Fallopian tubes I have seen without any aperture or fimbriated extremity, from a defect in the original formation, and terminating in a cul-de-sac.

Under such circumstances they were incapable of performing their office as a subservient to generation.

An Ovum in the Fallopian Tube

The Fallopian tube is sometimes dilated into a bag containing an ovum. This arises from the ovum being stopped in its progress from the ovarium to the uterus. When it is so stopped it does not die, but is gradually evolved as if it had been lodged in the cavity of the uterus. This, among many others, is a proof that the uterus is not the only organ which is fitted to evolve an ovum, but that other parts of the body can perform this office. While the ovum is enlarging, the Fallopian tube is more and more dilated, forming a thin bag round the ovum. The blood vessels passing to the ovarium, and the Fallopian tube where the ovum is contained are, gradually enlarged, in proportion to the increase of the ovum, in order to supply it with a sufficient quantity of blood. While this process is going on in the Fallopian tube, the uterus increases in bulk so as to be fully twice its natural size, and becomes more vascular. The cavity of its fundus is also lined with a membrana decidua, and the cervix uteri is plugged up with jelly. The uterus therefore undergoes a variety of changes, exactly similar to what takes place in natural pregnancy, being thrown into this mode of action from the original stimulus of impregnation. The ovum sometimes makes considerable progress in the Fallopian tube, and has been known to advance even to the full period of gestation; but more commonly it dies at an early period. In the course of the evolution of the ovum, the Fallopian tube has been known to rupture, and the person to die from internal haemorrhage. A very clear and accurate account of such a case has been published by Dr. Clarke, in the Medical and Chirurgical Transactions (109).

Hard Tumour growing from a Fallopian Tube

I have seen a hard round tumour growing from the outer surface of one of the Fallopian tubes. This when cut into exhibited precisely the same appearance of structure as the tubercle which grows from the surface of the uterus, viz. it consisted of a hard white substance, which was intersected by strong membranous septa. This, however, I believe to be a very rare appearance of disease.

Diseased appearances of the round Ligaments

The round ligaments partake of the inflammation of the uterus, when it is considerable, and has spread to its appendages. They are also, doubtless, subject to other diseases, but these are very rare, and have not fallen under my own observation, nor do I know of their having been particularly taken notice of by authors.

SYMPTOMS

The symptoms which attend the different morbid changes of the Fallopian tubes are at present not known; and they must, from the circumstances belonging to them, be very difficult to ascertain.

109. See p. 261. Vol. 2.

CHAPTER XXII

DISEASED APPEARANCES OF THE VAGINA

Inflammation of the Vagina

THE internal surface of the vagina, near the outward opening, is frequently inflamed, especially from the application of the venereal poison, but this hardly ever becomes the subject of examination after death.

Adhesion of the Sides of the Vagina

A very violent inflammation has sometimes been known to take place in the vagina, which has terminated in the mutual adhesion of the sides of the cavity. This adhesion is sometimes extended over a great part of the cavity, but I believe is often more confined, producing a stricture in some one part.

Ulcers of the Vagina

Ulcerations are not unusual in the vagina. They sometimes appear like spots of the internal surface, removed as it were by a knife, and sometimes there is a foul ragged ulcer. When this last is the case in any considerable degree, the ulcer has commonly not originated in the vagina, but has spread to it from the womb. When the ulcer spreads very much, communications are often made with the neighbouring parts, producing a most miserable state of existence. Thus communications are sometimes formed between the vagina and the rectum, or the vagina and the bladder.

Scirrhous Tumours in the Vagina

Scirrhous tumours occasionally arise in the vagina itself (although, I believe, rarely) when the uterus is unaffected. When cut into, they exhibit the usual scirrhous structure which has been often described.

Inversion of the Vagina

One of the most common diseases of the vagina is its inversion, or prolapsus: this is more apt to happen where the natural formation of the pelvis is large, where the external opening at the vulva is wide, and where the parts are generally relaxed. The prolapsus is more or less in different cases; in some the uterus does not pass out at the external parts, and in others the inversion of the vagina is complete, at the extremity of which is situated the os uteri. The protrusion has then different shapes; it sometimes forms a large rounded mass, and sometimes it is narrower and more elongated, extending, perhaps, five inches from the surface of the body. When this last has been the case, it has been sometimes mistaken for that species of monstrous formation called hermaphrodite. We may here take an opportunity of mentioning, that although in some of the common quadrupeds a real hermaphrodite structure has occasionally been found, yet it has hardly ever occurred in the human subject (110). When the vagina has been

110. Although the examples of what have been called hermaphrodites in the human species have, when strictly examined been hitherto found to belong to the male or the female sex; yet Dr. Storer of Nottingham has favoured me with an account of a person so strongly marked as a hermaphrodite, that no doubt can, I think, be reasonably entertained of this being the case. The person to whom this singular monstrosity belongs, is still alive, and has been carefully examined by Dr. Storer and other medical gentlemen, very able to judge concerning it; I shall therefore take the liberty of inserting, here, the account which Dr. Storer was so obliging as to send me.

The person bears a woman's name, and wears the apparel of a woman. She has a remarkable masculine look, with plain features, but no beard. She had never menstruated; and on this account she was desired by the lady with whom she lived as a servant, to become an out-patient at the Nottingham Hospital. At this time she was twenty four years of age, and had not been sensible of any bad health, but only came to the hospital in order to comply with the wishes of her mistress. Various medicines were tried without effect, which led to the suspicion of the hymen being imperforated, and the menstrual blood having accumulated behind it. She was, therefore, examined by Mr. Wright, one of the surgeons to the hospital, and by Dr. Storer.

The vagina was found to terminate in a cul-de-sac, two inches from the external surface of the labia. The head of the clitoris, and the external orifice of the meatus urinae, appeared as in the natural structure of a female, but there were no nymphae. The labia were more pendulous than usual, and contained each of them a body resembling a testicle of a moderate size, with its chord. The mammae resembled those of a woman. The person had no desire or partiality whatever for either sex.

long subject to inversion, its inner surface becomes in many parts harder; it is apt to be occasionally inflamed from external irritation, which not uncommonly advances to ulceration.

In inversion of the vagina and prolapsus of the uterus, if the cavity of the pelvis be examined, the fundus only of the uterus can be seen with its appendages very imperfectly, or the whole of the uterus is hid entirely: the bladder then appears to be in contact with the rectum. In this state of the uterus and its appendages, I have known adhesions formed between them and the neighbouring parts. These must have rendered the reduction of the uterus and the vagina into their natural situation very difficult, and perhaps, till the adhesions were a good deal elongated, impossible.

The Vagina very short

The vagina is sometimes very short. I have seen it, not more than half its natural length. This is an original defect in the formation of the part, and can only be ascertained by an examination.

The Vagina widened

The vagina is sometimes very much stretched or widened by large tumours which are lodged in it: these are chiefly polypi; and when they have been removed by art, the vagina, if it has not been for a long time stretched, recovers nearly its natural size.

The Vagina very narrow

The vagina has occasionally been found to be very much contracted with regard to its transverse diameter, from a defect in the original formation. This, however, occurs very rarely, and may in some degree be remedied by art.

SYMPTOMS

The symptoms which attend inflammation of the inner membrane of the vagina, and the labia, are too well known to require any description.

An adhesion of the sides of the vagina can only be distinctly known by an examination. It may, however, be strongly suspected where there has been a previous violent inflammation of the vagina, and since that period there has been no menstrual discharge, together with an unfitness for the usual intercourse between the sexes. When the adhesion has extended over a considerable part of the vagina, it is hardly possible by an operation to separate the adhering surfaces, and to restore the original canal. I have known attempts of this kind to fail in the most skillful hands; and it requires much nicety of management to avoid making an opening into the bladder or the rectum. Where the extent of the adhesion is small, it is very capable of being remedied by an operation, except perhaps very near the internal extremity of the vagina. As it is impossible, when the adhesion is complete, to know, *a priori,* whether it be of large or of small extent, it is almost always proper to attempt an operation; but this should only be done by a surgeon who is dexterous in the management of the knife, and with extreme caution. When there is merely a narrow line of adhesion, this may probably be discovered by the accumulation of the menstrual blood behind it; and it is possible that this accumulation may at length break through the adhesion and render an operation unnecessary. It would be absurd however, to put off an operation which under such circumstances must be very slight, for the very uncertain chance of this effect taking place.

Ulcers in the vagina can only be determined with accuracy by an examination of that passage in the living body. They are attended with more or less pain, and with a discharge of pus; but both of these symptoms belong also to inflammation of the vagina, without any ulceration whatever.

An inversion of the vagina is attended with a sense of bearing down (as patients commonly express it,) and a tumour passes outwards through the vulva, more especially in an erect posture. The exact circumstances of the disease can only be ascertained by an examination in the living body.

The existence of tumours growing in the vagina can only be accurately ascertained by an attentive examination.

CHAPTER XXIII

DISEASED AND PRETERNATURAL APPEARANCES OF THE EXTERNAL PARTS

The Hymen imperforated

THE hymen is sometimes found without a perforation in it, so that the vagina is completely shut up at its external extremity. This is an original malformation, which is frequently not discovered till the age of puberty, when the menstrual blood is accumulated behind it. It is of little consequence, as it can be easily remedied by a slight operation.

The Clitoris enlarged

An enlarged clitoris is also a natural deformity, less common than the other, but a more unfortunate one. At birth, the clitoris in such a case is often larger than the penis of a male child of the same age. It has a well formed prepuce and glans together with a fissure at its extremity, so as to resemble almost exactly the external appearance of the male organs. These cases have given rise to a mistake, with regard to the sex, and females have been often baptized for males. On most occasions, however, where there is an enlarged clitoris, the sex may be determined by the following circumstances. The labia are well formed, and when handled, no round bodies are felt in them, like the testicles. The fissure at the extremity of the glans does not lead to any canal of the urethra; but under the glans, and at the posterior extremity of the fissure, there is an opening which leads immediately to the bladder. I should believe, that by putting a small straight probe into this orifice, and passing it into the bladder, it could be at once determined, on most occasions, whether the child was male or female (111). If the child should live to grow up, the

111. Supposing the child to be a female, the probe will pass readily through a short straight canal; but supposing it to be a male, the probe will neither pass in a straight direction, nor without some degree of curvature being given to its shape, and the canal will be found to be of a considerable length.

clitoris enlarges, but, I believe, not in the same proportion as the penis would do. Such cases have been often mistaken for hermaphrodites.

The Nymphae enlarged

The nymphae are not uncommonly enlarged beyond their natural size. This sometimes happens to one only, and sometimes to both. When the nymphae are very much enlarged, they pass considerably beyond the surface of the body, and have the same sort of covering with the labia, losing by their exposure the fine, vascular, sensible covering of the natural nymphae. This is a monstrous formation of no great consequence, unless the enlargement be excessive, and even then the nymphae can be extirpated by art.

The external Labia growing together

The two external labia are sometimes united together by a fine line or junction, at the upper end of which are situated the meatus urinae, and the glans of the clitoris. This sort of monstrous formation is not at all common, and is very easily remedied. When the external labia are separated by a slight operation, all the parts behind are found perfect.

The two labia are sometimes joined together by a continuation of the common skin, so that the appearance of labia is lost entirely. This defect may also be remedied by art, and the parts within will be found to be well formed.

The external parts, particularly the inside of the nymphae, and the vestibulum, are subject to inflammation and ulcers from common causes, and especially from the application of the venereal poison. These diseases, although they are very often the subject of solicitude during life, yet are seldom examined after death, and therefore we shall omit them here altogether.

It is unnecessary to subjoin any account of symptoms to this chapter.

CHAPTER XXIV

DISEASED APPEARANCES OF THE BRAIN AND ITS MEMBRANES

Inflammation of the Dura Mater

THE dura mater is sometimes found in a state of inflammation. When this is the case, many extremely fine vessels, filled with florid blood, are seen in the inflamed portion of it, which pass between the dura mater and the cranium. These fine vessels are seldom so crowded as in most other parts of the body when inflamed, which arises from the nature of the membrane itself. In its natural state there are few blood vessels ramifying through it; and therefore, when it is inflamed, it does not appear so much crowded with vessels as other parts do which are naturally more vascular. Still, however, a person well acquainted with the natural appearance of the dura mater would be as much struck with the difference of its appearance when inflamed, as he would be with that of any other part of the body.

The dura mater during a state of inflammation sometimes forms a layer of coagulable lymph, which adheres upon its inner surface like an adventitious membrane; but this is very uncommon.

When the dura mater is inflamed, adhesions are sometimes formed between it and the other membranes of the brain, so that for a considerable extent they adhere together; but this appearance of disease is also very rare. The reason why diseased adhesions between the membranes of the brain are rare, depends, probably, upon coagulable lymph being seldom thrown out upon their surface when they are inflamed. This may be considered as a kind of peculiarity belonging to the membranes of the brain, for they bear some analogy to the membranes which line the circumscribed cavities of the body, and these last most commonly thrown out coagulable lymph upon their surface during inflammation.

It is not unusual when the dura mater has been inflamed, especially in consequence of some external violence, for suppuration to take place, and pus to be found covering a portion of the membrane.

The dura mater is likewise sometimes eroded by ulceration, but this is by no means frequent: it is more common, in violent injuries of the head, for a portion of it to become mortified.

Scrofulous Tumours connected with the Dura Mater

Scrofulous tumours are sometimes formed which are connected with the dura mater, but this happens very rarely. These resemble precisely the structure of a scrofulous absorbent gland, and occasionally there is found in them a curdly pus.

Spongy Tumours growing from the Dura Mater

Spongy tumours also grow from the dura mater, but they are very uncommon. Such tumours, as far as I have had an opportunity of examining them, are pulpy to the touch, and of a distinct, fibrous structure.

Bony Matter formed in the Dura Mater

One of the most common diseased appearances of the dura mater, is the formation of bony laminae in some part of it. These are usually very small, being not larger than the nail of a finger, but they are also occasionally of a much larger size. They are thin, and frequently very irregular in their edge. They are not to be found indifferently in every part of the dura mater, but are almost always adhering at the superior longitudinal sinus, or its falciform process. In some of them the proportion of the earth to the animal part is larger than in common bone.

There is often one of these ossifications only; but sometimes there are more of them. The falciform process has been said to be occasionally found almost entirely converted into bone; but this last appearance is very rare.

Very strong Adhesions of the Dura Mater to the Cranium

There is at all times a strong adhesion between the dura mater and the inside of the cranium. This adhesion is principally formed by small blood vessels which pass from the one to the other, and likewise by a close application of the fibrous structure of the membrane to the bone. In a natural state, however, the dura mater can be perfectly separated from the cranium; yet it sometimes happens that the adhesion is so strong, as to render it impossible to separate the two completely. The dura mater in such an attempt is torn in different parts into two laminae, one of which adheres to the bone, and the other lies upon the pia mater. Whether this preternatural strength of adhesion arises from a previous state of inflammation in the dura mater, or from some other cause I cannot determine; but it is not at all an uncommon appearance.

Diseased appearances of the Tunica Arachnoides

Diseased appearances of structure are very rare in the tunica arachnoides, and have almost been entirely overlooked by writers. The only diseased appearance of this coat, which I have observed, is that of its becoming a good deal thicker than it is naturally, so as to be a tolerably firm membrane. In this, as well as in its natural state, no blood vessels are to be seen ramifying upon it; or at least they are extremely few. It is also separated at some distance from the pia mater, by a serous fluid being interposed between the one and the other.

Diseased Appearances of the Pia Mater

Veins of the Pia Mater turgid with Blood

The most common diseased appearance of the pia mater is that of its veins being turgid with blood. This depends upon some impediment to the free return of the blood from the head towards the heart, which may arise from a variety of causes, and is very different from an inflamed state of the pia mater. The smaller branches of its arteries, filled with a florid blood, are not more numerous in this state than is natural, but its veins are much more distended with a dark blood.

The Pia Mater inflamed

When the pia mater is inflamed, it is upon the whole more difficult to distinguish this from its natural appearance than any other part of the body in the same condition. This depends upon the great number of very small vessels which naturally ramify upon it. In inflammation of the pia mater, these small vessels are much more numerous than in its natural state, are filled with a florid blood, and form by their anastomosis a beautiful net-work. It does not frequently occur, when the pia mater is inflamed, that it becomes so uniformly red as to shew no interstices between its vessels, a circumstance which happens in the inflammation of some other parts. The processes arising from the under surface of the pia mater are more crowded with vessels than usual, and there is a stronger adhesion between them and the substance of the brain.

It very rarely happens that any layer of coagulable lymph is formed in the inflammation of the pia mater which is so very common in inflammation of the pleura and the peritonaeum. When the pia mater is inflamed to a high degree, pus is formed: I have seen it effused over the whole upper surface of the brain, in consequence of an inflammation of the pia mater.

Close adhesions, for some considerable extent of surface, have been seen between the pia and dura mater, which are probably the consequence of inflammation; but these are very rare, and have not fallen under my own observation.

Scrofulous Tumours adhering to the Pia Mater

I have seen a number of scrofulous tumours adhering to the inside of the pia mater. They exhibit the true scrofulous structure, which has been often explained, and are very uncommon.

Air in the Vessels of the Pia Mater

It is not unusual to find some of the vessels of the pia mater filled with air. This may be generated by putrefaction, but it is also sometimes seen when no process of this kind appears to have taken place. Under such circumstances, it is probable that air is extricated by some new arrangement in the constituent parts of the blood.

Hydatids

Little cysts (112) containing water (which are generally called hydatids,) have been seen adhering to the pia mater; but this is a very rare appearance of disease.

A Part of the Pia Mater bony

It occasionally happens, although I believe very seldom, that a portion of the pia mater is converted into bone. It has not occurred to me to observe such a change of structure in this membrane, but Dr. Soemmerring mentions that a specimen of this disease is preserved in his collection.

Diseased Appearances in the Substance of the Brain – Inflammation

The substance of the brain, under which I include both the cerebrum and cerebellum, is liable to inflammation, although it is not common, when no external injury has been applied to the head. When inflammation takes place, it is rarely extended over any large portion of the brain, but is rather confined to one or more distinct parts of it. In this state of disease the inflamed portion becomes of a red colour, although this is seldom very intense. When cut into, the colour is found to arise from a great many small vessels, which are filled with blood. If the inflamed portion be upon the surface of the brain, the membranes in the neighbourhood are also commonly inflamed. The part which is inflamed has no peculiar hardness, but yields nearly the same sensation to the touch, as it would do in a healthy state.

---

112. Vid. Lieutaud, Tom. II. p. 145.

Abscesses

Inflammation of the brain frequently advances to suppuration, and abscesses are formed in it. When these are of a large size, the weight of the pus breaks down the structure of the neighbouring parts, and they look simply as if they had been destroyed, or very much injured by the pressure. When the abscesses are small, there is an ulcerated appearance of the cavity in which the pus is contained.

Gangrene

Portions of the brain occasionally become gangrenous, especially after violent injuries of the head; but I believe this appearance of disease is extremely rare, where an inflammation of the brain has taken place from any other cause. I have met, however, with one instance of this; a portion of the brain at the inflamed part was of a very dark brown colour, and as soft as the most rotten pear.

The Brain very soft

It is extremely common, when the brain is examined in a person who has been dead for several days, to find such a softness of its substance, that it can hardly admit of being cut so as to leave a smooth surface, and the smallest pressure of the fingers breaks it down into a pultaceous mass. The brain, however, will sometimes retain, for several days, the firmness and resistance which it had during life; yet this is by no means common. Neither of these appearances is to be considered as produced by disease.

Sometimes, however, a part of the medullary substance of the brain becomes morbidly soft, and loses its natural texture, acquiring nearly the consistence of a custard. Dr. John Hunter, physician to the army, has observed this in the medulla of the hemispheres of the brain, near the lateral ventricles. He has met with this appearance in cases of fatuity, where the persons were advanced in life, and also combined with effusions of blood in apoplexy.

The Brain very firm

The brain is sometimes found to be considerably firmer than in its healthy state, to be tougher, and to have a greater degree of elasticity than usual; it will bear to be pulled out with some force, and will readily re-act so as to restore itself, or when pressed will recover its former shape. Under such circumstances the ventricles are sometimes found to be enlarged in size, and full of water. The brain has even been said to become so hard and dry as to be friable between the fingers; and the medullary substance, in these cases, is represented as being much lighter than in a natural state. It is probable, however, that these accounts are a good deal exaggerated. It has been remarked that in such cases the cerebellum is very often unaffected.

A white firm Substance formed in the Brain

It is not very unusual to see a white substance formed in the brain of a uniform smooth texture, and possessing a considerable degree of hardness. The brain adheres to this substance, and round its edge appears often more vascular than usual. The substance is scrofulous in its nature, for I have had an opportunity of seeing it converted into a scrofulous pus. There are frequently more than one of these substances formed in the brain at a time.

It is also not unusual to find rounded masses of the same sort of substance, lying as it were imbedded in the brain, or in its interstices; some of these I have seen as large as a walnut. When such tumours are formed, it happens frequently that there is an increased quantity of water in the lateral ventricles of the brain.

Encysted Tumours and Hydatids

Encysted tumours containing a serous fluid (113) have sometimes been found in the substance of the brain; but they have never come under my own observation, and are very uncommon.

In one instance I have known hydatids to be accumulated in the

113. Vid. Li eutaud, Tom. II. p. 194, 195.

lateral ventricules of the brain, but this is still a more uncommon appearance of disease than the other. They seemed to be of the same nature with hydatids of the liver (114).

Bony Tumours pressing upon the Brain

Bony tumours are sometimes formed in the cranium, which press upon a part of the brain. They most commonly consist of an irregular mass, which is formed of bony processes, with a fleshy substance filling up the interstices between them. Of this sort of tumour there are several examples of Dr. Hunter's collection.

It has sometimes happened, but very rarely, that all the bones of the cranium have become extremely thickened, and have encroached, by their growth, upon the cavity which contains the brain. Of this there is a remarkable specimen in Mr. Hunter's collection, where the bones of the cranium are at least three times as thick as in the natural state. They are also, in the case to which I allude, much more spongy than usual in their texture.

A nodule of a substance having the appearance of ivory, has also been known to be formed in the bones of the cranium, and to protrude considerably into its cavity. This too occurs very rarely, but a specimen of it is preserved in Mr. Hunter's collection. Whatever may be the variety in the morbid processes which produce these changes of structure in the bones of the cranium, their effects upon the functions of the brain must be nearly the same, as they form a permanent cause of compression.

Bony Ridges irritating the Brain

Upon the inner surface of the basis of the cranium there is always some irregularity. This consists in numerous ridges and small eminences with depressed surfaces interposed between them. It happens occasionally that there is a morbid growth of these eminences and ridges, forming sharp spicula and sharp edges of bone. These run into the brain, and irritate very violently the nervous system.

114. This case was communicated to me by Mr. Burnall, who attended the patient, and examined the appearances after death.

Hydrocephalus

One of the most common appearances of disease in the brain, is the accumulation of water in its ventricles (115); this generally takes place when a child is very young, and even sometimes before birth. The water is accumulated in greater or less quantity in different cases. It sometimes amounts only to a few ounces, and occasionally to many pints. When the quantity of water is very considerable, the fornix is raised at its anterior extremity in consequence of its accumulation, and an immediate opening of communication is thereby formed between the lateral ventricles (116). From this cause too a part of the water passes very readily into the third ventricle, and from thence into the fourth. The water is of a purer colour, and more limpid, than what is found in dropsy of the thorax or abdomen. It appears, however, to be generally of the same nature with the water that is accumulated in both of those large cavities. In some trials which I have made, it partly coagulated upon the application of the common acids, exactly like the water in hydrothorax and ascites, or like the serum of the blood. But there is much variety in the quantity of the coagulable matter. In some instances the water in

115. Mr. Home has known an instance where water was accumulated in large quantity in the third ventricle, and had forced its way between the fine laminae of the medullary substance which compose the septum lucidum, without escaping into either of the lateral ventricles. This may be said to be a new situation of hydrocephalus, and is of very rare occurrence.

116. A distinguished author has, in a late publication, insisted very strongly upon the existence of an immediate communication between the two lateral ventricles of the brain, and has expressed great surprise that it has been denied by several teachers of anatomy in London. Without entering into any dispute about this matter, which in itself is of no great importance, I shall briefly mention what appears to me to be the real state of the circumstances. The fornix at its anterior extremity lies loose upon a part of the thalami nervorum opticorum, and there is a small chink on each side of the fornix leading obliquely downwards from the lateral ventricle to the anterior extremity of the third ventricle. While the fornix is allowed to remain in its natural situation, there seems to be no immediate communication between the lateral ventricles. But when the fornix is elevated (which may be very easily done) then the lateral ventricles communicate directly with each other; and the communication is more or less according to the degree of the elevation. It may be said, that the lateral ventricles still communicate together by means of the third ventricle. This, however, is not properly an immediate communication between the two lateral ventricles, unless any two cavities which communicate with a third, may be properly said to communicate directly or immediately with each other.

hydrocephalus contains a very small proportion of coagulable matter, and in others it is almost entirely free from it.

When water is accumulated in the ventricles to a very large quantity, the substance of the brain, especially upon the sides and at the upper surface, appears almost to be a sort of pulpy bag, containing a fluid. The scull too upon such occasions is very much enlarged in size, and altered in its shape. The cranium is exceedingly large in proportion to the size of the face. The projections are very considerable at the centres of ossification, from whence the frontal, parietal, and occipital bones were originally formed, and the membranous divisions between these several bones are very wide. When the scalp is removed, so as to give an opportunity of looking immediately upon the cranium, the bones are found to be very thin, often not thicker than a shilling, and there are frequently broad spots of membrane in the bone. The reason of this last appearance is, that ossification takes place in many points of the membrane in such cases in order to make a quicker progress, but the water accumulates too rapidly for it, so that spots of membrane are left not converted into bone. When such appearances take place in hydrocephalus, the disease has been of long continuance, occasionally for some years.

Water upon the Surface of the Brain, and between its Membranes

Water is also sometimes formed under the pia mater, and upon the surface of the brain, but very rarely in any considerable quantity. There is, generally, at the same time, a greater quantity than natural in the ventricles.

Water is likewise found in small quantity between the dura and pia mater.

It is related by authors, that water has been formed occasionally between the dura mater and the cranium (117). From the nature of the adhesion between the cranium and this membrane one would not easily be led to suspect an accumulation of water between them, and such cases are at least to be considered as very uncommon.

117. Vid. Lieutaud, Tom. II. p. 229, 230.

Blood effused or extravasated

Blood is frequently found effused within the cavity of the cranium in various situations. It may either be poured out by the rupture of some vessel in the substance of the brain itself, or into some of the ventricles. It is frequently effused upon the surface of the brain, or upon some of its membranes. This is most apt to happen where the effusion is in consequence of external violence.

The quantity of blood which is effused from the rupture of vessels in the brain is frequently very considerable. It is commonly found in a coagulated state, and the texture of the brain in the neighborhood is often very much hurt from the pressure. Blood is not equally liable to be effused into every part of the substance of the brain. Where an effusion has taken place without external injury, it is almost constantly found in the medullary part of one of the hemispheres, and often near the lateral ventricles, so that a quantity of blood has at the same time escaped into one or both of these cavities. It sometimes happens that the brain is very soft in its consistence at the place of this effusion, a remark which has been made by Dr. John Hunter.

When blood is extravasated within the cavity of the cranium from some external injury, the vascular system is usually sound, except for the rupture which may have happened. But when extravasation happens within the cavity of the cranium, without internal injury, the vascular system of the brain is almost always diseased. It is very common in examining the brains of persons who are considerably advanced in life, to find the trunks of the internal carotid arteries upon the side of the sella turcica very much diseased, and this disease extends frequently more or less into the small branches. The disease consists in a bony or earthy matter being deposited in the coats of the arteries, by which they lose a part of their contractile and distensile powers, as well as of their tenacity. The same sort of diseased structure is likewise found in the basilary artery and its branches.

The vessels of the brain under such circumstances of disease, are much more liable to be ruptured than in a healthy state. Whenever blood is accumulated in unusual quantity, or the circulation is going on in them with unusual vigour, they are liable to this accident, and accordingly in either of these states, extravasations of blood frequently happen. Were the internal carotid arteries and the basilary artery not subject to the diseased alteration of structure which we have described, effusions of blood within the cavity of the cranium, where there has been no previous external injury, would probably be much more rare.

Cavities in the Brain containing a serous Fluid

Cavities containing a serous fluid are sometimes observed in the substance of the brain. They almost constantly occur in the medullary part of the hemispheres, and the substance of the brain immediately surrounding these cavities is tough and smooth, so as to resemble a membrane. They would appear to be the remains of the cavities formed by extravasated blood, in cases of apoplexy, where the patients have lived afterwards for some months or years. The extravasated blood would seem in such cases to have been dissolved, and taken up by absorption; but the injury is not repaired, and a cavity remains afterwards filled with a serous fluid (118).

Aneurysm of the internal Carotid Arteries on the Side of the Sella Turcica

The internal carotid arteries are very apt, in persons of an advanced age, to become ossified, and the same morbid changes may be traced along their branches. It occurs, however, very rarely, that they are distended at any part into an aneurysmal sack, like the arteries in some other parts of the body. I have been informed of an instance of this kind, where both the internal carotid arteries, on the side of the sella turcica, were distended into a little aneurysm (119). One of these aneurysms was about

---

118. I had an opportunity of observing, lately, a well marked case of this sort, in a person who had had several attacks of the apoplexy, and at length was cut off by one of them. Dr. John Hunter has observed a good many instances of it, and a case occurred some years ago to Mr. Wilson, lecturer on anatomy, whose accuracy is well known, where the cavity which remained was of a very large size.

119. I owe my acquaintance with this case to Dr. Blane.

the size of a cherry and the other was somewhat smaller. It is remarkable that in the only two instances which have come to my knowledge, of aneurysms being formed in the arteries of the head and brain, there has been an aneurysm in both arteries in the same situation, and at the same time. I once met with an aneurysm in each of the carotid arteries at the origin of the internal carotids, and in the case just described, there was an aneurysm in each of the two internal carotid arteries upon the side of the sella turcica.

Diseased Appearances of the Plexus Choroides
Little Bags in the Plexus Choroides

The most common diseased appearance of the plexus choroides is that of little round transparent bags, which adhere to it, and which have commonly been called hydatids. These are generally about the size of a garden pea, but sometimes, they have been seen as large as a gooseberry. From several examinations which I have made of them, they would seem to be formed by a distension of the vein which runs along the edge of the plexus choroides. I have been able to distend them fully with air, by making an opening into this vein, and inflating air into it through a small blowpipe.

Round Tumours adhering to the Plexus Choroides

Tumours sometimes adhere to the plexus choroides. These are small in their size, or a round shape, and occur but rarely. They seem to be the same kind with the round tumours which are sometimes found imbedded in the brain, and I believe are scrofulous.

Diseased Appearances of the Pineal Gland
Earthy Matter in the Pineal Gland

A little earthy matter is almost constantly found in the pineal gland. It is sometimes in very small quantity, but not unfrequently the quantity is very considerable. The particles of the earth do not adhere strongly together, but are easily separable by pressure between the fingers. The existence of a small quantity of earth is so common in the pineal gland, that it cannot well be considered as a disease. I think, however, that in some instances I have found this gland without any deposition of earthy matter.

Pineal Gland said to be scirrhous

The pineal gland has been mentioned by authors as being sometimes scirrhous. I have felt it on some occasions a little firmer than on others; but it has never occurred to me to observe that alteration of structure in it, which could be properly called scirrhous, and I believe it to be a very rare disease.

Water in the Pineal Gland

The pineal gland has been found to be very much distended with a limpid water (120); but this too is very uncommon.

Diseased Appearances of the Pituitary Gland

This gland is very little liable to be affected by disease. It has only occurred to me to observe in it one morbid change. It was, in that case, enlarged to twice its natural size, and was converted into a substance, possessing an obscurely fibrous structure.

Diseased Appearances of the Nerves

It rarely happens that any of the nerves within the cavity of the cranium appear diseased. I have, however, sometimes seen a nerve a good deal smaller in its size than it ought to be, softer in its texture, and of a less opaque colour; this I recollect to have been particularly the case with one of the optic nerves in a person who was blind of one eye (121).

---

120. Vid. Morgagni, Epist. LXII. Art. 15.

121. I have seen an instance of a considerable tumour being formed in a nerve. The tumour was very solid in its texture, of a yellowish white colour, and larger in its size than a goose's egg. The nerve seemed to be in some measure lost in the tumour, and in one part of it a fibrous structure could be observed pretty distinctly, similar to that of a nerve. This swelling occurred in one of the auxillary nerves, and was extirpated by Mr. Home, at St. George's Hospital.

Mal-formations of the Brain

These are the principal diseased changes which take place in the brain and its appendages. I have just to add, that the brain is subject to a great variety from original monstrous formation. A great part of what is usually called the cerebrum is sometimes wanting, while the cerebellum, and the medulla spinalis are entire; sometimes there is hardly any vestige of either the cerebrum or cerebellum, and the medulla spinalis is very much diminished in size; at other times there is a total want of the brain, and there is no appearance of the medulla spinales. In this case one should expect a want of nerves through the whole body. It is, however, not so; nerves are found distributed in the common way, through the limbs, and the dorsal nerves can be seen arising from a membrane somewhat resembling the dura mater in the canal behind the vertebrae. When there is a total want of brain, it sometimes happens that there is a medulla spinalis, which, however, is of a very small size. In cases of deficiency in the brain, the cranium is nearly upon a level with the two eyes, and there is often upon the scalp a soft, spongy escrescence. This is generally divided into distinct protuberant masses, and is covered with a fine skin, capable of being rendered very vascular by injection. When cut into, the spongy excrescence consists of pretty large cells, which are filled with a sort of grumous matter.

There is also frequently, instead of this excrescence, a bag growing from the skin of the scalp, and passing downwards so as to cover more or less of the back of the trunk. This bag sometimes consists of a fine membrane, with little strength; and sometimes it is rather thick, with considerable firmness. It sometimes communicates with the cavity of the cranium by a considerable opening; and sometimes the communication is very small. It is filled with an aqueous fluid, and in some instances there is also in it a portion of the brain.

SYMPTOMS

Inflammation of the dura mater is not distinguished by any peculiar symptoms. The symptoms which belong to it, are the same with those which attend inflammation of the other membranes, and even differ but little from the symptoms which take place in inflammation of the brain itself. The symptoms are, pain in the head, delirium, symptomatic fever, and sometimes convulsive motions.

When tumours have been found adhering to the dura mater, or the other membranes of the brain, a long continued pain in the head has commonly been remarked, sometimes delirium, sometimes convulsions, and sometimes it has been said, the ordinary symptoms of apoplexy.

Where bony matter has been formed in the dura mater, with sharp processes growing from it, convulsive motions have very commonly occurred in various parts of the body, often a continued pain in the head, and sometimes delirium.

In cases where the veins of the pia mater have been found turgid with blood, stupor has very frequently occurred, sometimes delirium, and sometimes, it has been said even apoplexy in its perfect form.

The symptoms of inflammation in the pia mater, are the same with those which attend inflammation of the dura mater, and they have been already noticed.

In inflammation of the substance of the brain, there is pain in the head, delirium, symptomatic fever, and sometimes coma.

Where an abscess has been formed in the brain, pain, delirium, and coma, have been remarked, sometimes a paralysis of a part of the body, and sometimes convulsions. The last symptom has been observed most frequently to occur when the abscess has been formed in the tuberculum annulare or in the medulla oblongata, or in the neighbourhood of these structures so that the pus could affect them by its pressure.

The brain has sometimes been found more firm and elastic than is natural in cases of mania. I have been informed, however, lately, from the best authority, that this state of brain is not common in maniacs; and that in them it is generally not more firm, nor more elastic, than in people whose minds have always been sound.

The symptoms which have been observed to attend the formation of solid, or encysted tumours in the brain, are a permanent pain in the head, which is occasionally very violent, sometimes delirium, sometimes convulsions, and sometimes, it has been said, the common symptoms of apoplexy. It is worthy of remark here, that when tumours of any kind press upon the thalami nervorum opticorum, or the optic nerves themselves, within the cranium, vision generally becomes impaired in various ways (122); and that when tumours press upon the tuberculum annulare, or the medulla oblongata, convulsions are very apt to occur.

In the case where hydatids were accumulated in the lateral ventricle, the person had been subject for a long time to pain in his head, which was often violent, and towards the close of the disease, had several convulsion-fits, in one of which he expired. Neither his sight nor hearing were impaired.

The symptoms of hydrocephalus, are a pain in the head, stupor, convulsive motions, picking of the nose, grinding of the teeth during sleep, occasional flushings of the face, and towards the latter end of the disease, a dilatation of the pupils and squinting. The stomach is commonly affected with sickness, and the bowels are with difficulty acted upon by purgative medicines. In the beginning of this disease the pulse is frequent but regular; when the disease has made a further progress, it is slow and irregular; and towards the latter end of the disease, it becomes again more regular and frequent. When the progress of the disease has been very gradual, and the patient has continued to live for some months, or even years, the functions of the brain have been found in many instances, to be less impaired than might have been expected, till near its close.

Where blood has been effused upon any of the membranes of the brain, the patient is more or less in a comatose state, according to the degree of the effusion, or the different susceptibility of the brain in different individuals to be affected by pressure. Innumerable instances shew, that the brain will have its functions impaired in very different degrees, from the same apparent degree of injury.

When blood is effused into the substance of the brain, apoplexy

---

122. I have known one case in which the optic nerves at their junction were pressed by a tumour as large as a gooseberry, and yet the pupils were not dilated, nor the eyesight impaired, till within a day or two of the person's death. There was only a very violent pain in the fore part of the head.

is produced, which is attended with the following symptoms, viz. coma; often stertous breathing; a paralysis, commonly of one half of the body; and often convulsive motions. The pulse is slow, full, and generally very strong. When the patient is not cut off at once, but lives for some time after the attack, the hemiphlegia, which is almost constantly an effect of this disease, is generally upon the opposite side of the body from that of the brain, in which the effusion of blood has taken place. This would seem to shew, that the right side of the body derives its nervous influence from the left side of the brain, and the left side of the body its nervous influence from the right side of the brain. In a few instances, however, the hemiphlegia has occurred on the same side of the body with the effusion (123).

---

123. Dr. John Hunter has made some very accurate dissections relative to apoplexy, and its consequences, which formed the subject of the Gulstonian lectures, read by him, 1796, before the College of Physicians. By these lectures, I have been enabled to give a more satisfactory account of the appearances connected with this disease, than I should have been otherwise.

INDEX

A

Abscess
  bladder, 208
  brain, 271, 281
  heart, 83
  intestine, 139, 146-147, 154
  kidney, 198-199, 204, 205
  larynx, 114, 115, 127
  liver, 170, 171
  lungs, 104
  pancreas, 195, 197
  prostate, 223
  testicle, 234
  thymus, 125
  ureter, 199
  urethra, 227
Adhesion
  pericardium, 77-78, 81
  peritoneal, 132-133, 136, 151, 169-170, 181, 257
  pleural, 97, 99, 100-101
  tunica vaginalis, 233
  vagina, 260, 263
Alcoholism
  cirrhosis, 29, 172
Amelia, Princess, 12
Anatomic Theatre, 8, 9
Anencephaly, 280
Aneurysm
  aorta, 86-87, 93, 222
  berry, 277-278
  heart, 85-86, 93
Anomalies, Congenital
  see Congenital Anomalies
Anus
  fistula, 155, 156
  imperforate, 156
Aorta
  aneurysm, 86-87, 93, 122
  white spots, 87
Arsenic
  stomach, 138-139, 144
Arteriosclerosis
  aorta, 87
  coronary, 30, 88, 94
  cranial vessels, 276, 277
Ascites, 130, 135, 175, 190

B

Baillie, Dorothy, 7, 8
Baillie, James, 7
Baillie, Matthew, 5-33
  anatomic activities, 6
  atlas, 10, 32-36, 48-51 (editions)
  autobiography, 17
  birth, 7
  busts, 14
  death, 5, 14
  degrees, 9
  dissections, 11, 19, 45-46
  education, 7
  illness, 12
  lecturer, 9, 11
  library, 10-11
  medical practice, 11, 12
  miscellaneous papers, 11, 19, 44-45
  museum activities, 9, 10
  textbook, 5, 9, 10, 19, 23-27, 47, 53–283
  wife, 17
Baker, Sir George, 24
Balliol College, 7
Bell, Charles, 14
Bichat
  book, 5, 20
Bile Ducts, 182-183
  dilatation, 182
  obliteration, 183, 187
Bladder, 207-219
  abscesses, 208

calculus, 213-216, 218
cancer, 209
from rectum, 209
from uterus, 209
contracted, 216
distention, 216
diverticuli (cysts), 210
excrescences, 209, 218
exstrophy (anterior part wanting), 216-217
hernia, 217
inflammation, 207, 217, 220
lithotomy, 208
obstruction, 211
polypus, 209-210, 218
recto-vesicular fistula, 157, 208, 217
schirrhus, 208
symptoms, 217-219
thickening, 210-212
two chambers, 212, 218
ulcers, 208, 218
utero-vesicular fistula, 241
Brain, 266-283
abscesses, 271, 281
absence cerebrum, 280
anencephaly, 280
berry aneurysm, 277-278
bony tumors, 273
cavities, 277
enlarged ventricles, 272
firm, 272, 281
gangrene, 271
hemorrhage, 276, 282-283
hydatids, 272, 282
hydrocephalus, 274-275, 282
inflammation, 270
malformations, 280
membranes – *see* Brain, Coverings
meningocele, 280
post-mortem, 271
soft, 27
symptoms, 280-283
trauma, 271
tumor, 272, 273, 281
tumors choroid plexus, 278
Brain, Coverings, 266-270
adhesions, 266, 268
air vessels, 269-270
arachnoid thickening, 268
bony, 267, 270, 281
congestion (turgid), 268
hemorrhage, 276, 282
hydatids, 270
inflammation, 266, 269, 280, 281
meningocele, 280
scrofula, 263, 269
tumors, 267, 281
water, 275

C

Calculi
bladder, 213-216, 218
gall-stones, 181-182, 183-186, 188
intestine, 163
kidney, 199, 202-203, 206
level, 109, 111
pancreas, 195-196, 197
prostate, 225, 226
seminal vesicles, 222
spleen, 192
stomach, 144
thymus, 125
ureter, 202
urethra, 227-228
Caruncle
urethra, 229, 231
Charlotte, Princess, 12
Cirrhosis, 28, 35, 135
Clift, William, 32
Clossy, S., 23-24, 28
Congenital Anomalies, 22
bladder, 216
brain, 275, 280
gall-bladder, 187
genitalia, external, 264, 265
heart, 90-92
intestine, 150, 156
kidney, 203-204
ovary, 221, 255-256
pancreas, 196
pericardium, 20, 80-81
spleen, 193
testicle, 236-237
thyroid, 112-113, 126
urethra, 230
uterus, 247
Coronary Disease, 30, 88, 94

Cranium
  hydrocephalus, 275
  ivory nodules, 273
  ridges, 273
  thickened, 273
Croup
  larynx, 128
  trachea, 126, 128
Cruikshank, Mr., 9, 16, 123

D

Denmon, Dr., 8, 17
Dermoid Cyst, 253-254
Diabetes, 21
  kidney, 199-200, 206
  liver, 200
Diphtheria, *see* Croup
Diverticuli
  bladder, 210
  pharynx, 121-122
  stomach, 141
Duodenum
  inflammation, 183
  ulcer, 153
Duntisbourne Estate, 12
Dysentery, 154, 166

E

Emphysema, 29, 34
Empyema, 97-98, 101, 104
Esophagus, 118-120
  aphthae, 118
  bony, 114
  cartilaginous, 120
  hydrophobia, 139
  pharyngo-esophageal fistula, 121
  scrofula, 129
  stricture
    puckering, 119, 128
    spasmodic, 118, 128
    ulcer, 120, 128
  symptoms, 128-129
  ulcer, 113-114, 120-121, 124
Exstrophy Bladder, 216-217

F

Fallopian Tube, 257-259
  adhesions, 257
  hydrosalpinx (dropsy), 257-258
  inflammation, 257
  pregnancy, 258-259
  stricture (cul-de-sac), 258
  symptoms, 259
  tumors, 259
Fernel
  book, 5, 24, 28
Fistula
  anus, 155, 156
  cholecysto-gastric, 183
  pharyngo-esophageal, 121
  recto-prostatic, 224
  recto-vaginal, 157, 208, 260
  recto-vesicular, 157, 208, 217
  urethral, 221
  utero-vesicular, 241
  vagino-vesicular, 260
Fordyce, Dr., 8

G

Gall-Bladder, 181-188
  absent (wanting), 187
  adhesions, 181
  bile, 186-187
  bony, 182
  distended, 187
  gall-stones, 181-182, 183-186, 188
  gastric fistula (canal), 183
  hydatids, 187
  inflammation, 181, 187
  post-mortem, 185-186
  symptoms, 187-188
  ulcers, 181-182, 188
General Pathology, 26
Genitalia, External, Female, 264-265
  enlarged clitoris, 264-265
  enlarged nymphae, 263
  fused labia, 265
  hermaphrodite, 265
  imperforate hymen, 264
  inflammation, 265
  ulcers, 265
  venereal poison, 265
George III, 7
Glands, Absorbent, 123-124
  bony, 124, 164-165

cancerous, 164
scirrhous, 124
scrofula, 123-124, 164, 168
Glasgow, University, 7
Gold-Headed Cane, 5, 12, 17, 24

H

Heart, 83-95
abscesses, 83
aneurysm, 85-86, 93
endocardial cushion defect, 90-91
enlarged, 92, 95
hydatids, 93, 95
hypoplastic right heart, 90
inflammation, 83, 93
malformation, 90-92
mortified, 83
patent ductus arteriosus, 90
polypus, 84
rheumatism, 25
rupture, 86, 89
symptoms, 93-95
transposition great vessels, 91
ulcers, 83
valve disease, 36, 88-89, 94
ventricular septal defect, 91
white spots, 83-84
Heberden, William, 29
Hemopericardium, 89-90
Hemorrhoids, 155-156, 166
Hermaphrodite, 265
Hernias
diaphragmatic, 150
intestine, 149-153, 165
umbilical, 150
Home, Sir Everard, 16
Hunter, John, 5, 7, 8, 9
death, 10
Hunter, William, 5, 7, 8, 69
death, 9
Hunterian Oration, 16
Hydatids
brain, 272, 282
brain covering, 270
gall-bladder, 187
heart, 93, 95
intestine, 155
kidney, 201-202, 203, 205
liver, 175-177, 180
lung. 109, 111
peritoneum, 134, 136-137
spleen, 192, 194
testicle, 233, 238-239
uterus, 246-247, 250
Hydrocele, 232, 238
Hydrocephalus, 274-275, 282
Hydropericardium, 78, 81
Hydrosalpinx, 257-258
Hydrophobia
esophagus, 139
pharynx, 139
stomach, 139, 145
Hydrothorax – *see* Pericardium, dropsy
Hymen
imperforate, 264
Hypospadias, 230

I

Inflammation
bladder, 207, 217, 220
brain, 270
brain coverings, 266, 269, 280, 281
genitalia, external, 265
Fallopian tube, 259
gall-bladder, 181, 187
heart, 83, 93
intestine, 146, 151, 165
kidney, 198, 205
larynx, 115
liver, 170, 179
lungs, 103, 110
mesentery, 168
ovary, 251, 256
pericardium, 75-77, 81, 83
peritoneum, 131-132, 135-136, 146, 169, 178, 207, 240, 251
pleura, 96, 100, 103, 110
prostate, 223, 226
seminal vesicles, 220
spleen, 189-190, 193
stomach, 138-139, 144
testicle, 233-234, 239
thyroid, 112, 125
trachea, 115, 127
urethra, 228-229, 230
uterus, 240, 248

vagina, 260, 262-263
Intestine, 146-168
air, 161-162, 167
arsenic, 139
bony, 162-163
calculous, 163
cancer, 153-154
dysentery, 154, 166
fistula-in-ano, 155, 156
hernias (ruptures), 149-153, 165
diaphragmatic, 150
inguinal, 150, 152-153
umbilical, 150
imperforate anus (cul-de-sac), 156
inflammation, 146, 151, 165
intus-susceptio, 149, 165
mortification, 148, 151
perforation, 147
piles, 155-156, 166
polyps (thickened membranes), 155
post-mortem, 163
recto-vaginal fistula, 157, 208
recto-vesicular fistula, 157, 208, 217
schirrhus, 153-154, 166
small-pox, 163
strangulation, 165
symptoms, 165-168
ulcer, 139, 146-147, 154
worms, 157-161, 167
Intus-susceptio, 149, 165

J

Johnson, Samuel, 30

K

Kidney, 198-206
abscesses, 198-199, 204, 205
absent, 203, 204
anomalies (original varieties), 203-204
bony, 203
calculi, 199, 202-203, 206
cartilaginous, 205
diabetes, 199-200, 206
ectopic, 203
horseshoe (fused), 203
hydatids, 201-202, 203, 205
hypoplastic, 203
inflammation, 198, 205
scirrhus, 199, 205
scrofula, 198, 199, 204
soft, 200
symptoms, 205-206

L

Laennec, 16, 29
Larynx, 114-115
bony, 114, 127
croup, 128
inflammation, 115
scrofula, 115
symptoms, 127
ulcer, 114, 115, 127
Leiomyoma
uterus, 241-242, 249
Lithopedion, 245
Lithotomy, 208
Liver, 169-180
abscess, 170-171
alcohol, 172
cirrhosis (common tubercle), 171-172, 174, 179
cysts, earthy, 177
diabetes, 200
hard, 174, 179
hydatids, 175-177, 180
inflammation, 170, 179
mortification, 171
rupture, 177
schirrhus, 172
scrofula, 173-174, 186
soft, 174
symptoms, 178-180
tubercle, large white, 172, 179
worms, 178
Lungs
abscesses, 104
air cells enlarged, 107, 111
air distention, 107
air vesicles, 108
bone, 108-109
from knee tumor, 109
concretions, 109, 111
edema (water), 107
hydatids, 109, 111
inflammation, 103, 110
liver-like, 108, 111

phthisis, 106
post-mortem, 103-104
scrofula, 104
symptoms, 110-111
tubercles, 105-106, 110
tumor, 109
Lymph Nodes – *see* Glands, Absorbent

M

Mediastinum
anterior, 124-125
posterior, 115-124
Medical Chirurgical Society, 12
Meningocele, 280
Mesentery
fatty tumours, 165
inflammation, 168
Morgagni
book, 5, 20, 21, 22, 23, 28, 69
Museum, Baillie's
activities, 9-10
specimens, 40-43

N

Nerves
atrophy optic n., 279

O

Osborne, Dr., 8
Osler, William, 17
Ovary, 251-256
absence (wanting), 255-256
bony, 251-252
cysts (dropsy), 252, 256
dermoid (fatty), 253-254
enlarged, 252
inflammation, 251, 256
pregnancy, 255
scirrhus, 251, 256
scrofula, 252
shrinkage, 255
symptoms, 256
Oxford, 7, 8, 9

P

Pancreas, 195-197
abscess, 195, 197
absence, 196
calculi, 195-196, 197
hard, 195, 197
scirrhus, 183
symptoms, 196-197
Paraplegia, 20
Penis, 230
Pericardium, 75-83
absence, 20, 80-81
adhesions, 77-78, 81
air, 26
bony, 25, 81
dropsy, 78, 81
dry, 79-80, 82
hemopericardium, 89-90
inflammation, 75-77, 81, 83
pus, 76-77
scrofula, 79, 82
symptoms, 81-82
Peritoneum, 130-137
adhesions, 132-133, 136, 151, 169-170, 181, 257
ascites, 130, 135, 175, 190
bony, 162, 170
cartilaginous, 134
hydatids, 134, 136-137
inflammation, 131-132, 135-136, 146, 169, 178, 207, 240, 251
pneumoperitoneum (air), 134
scrofula, 133-134
symptoms, 135-137
tumors, 134
from stomach, 134
steatomatous, 134
Pharynx, 120-122
fungus, 120-121
hydrophobia, 139
pharyngo-esophageal fistula, 121
pouch, 121-122
scrofula, 121
ulcer, 121
Philosophical Transactions, 19
Phthisis, 106
Pineal
earthy matter, 278-279
scirrhous, 279
water, 279
Pitcairn, David, 5, 11, 24, 32

Pituitary
enlarged, 279
fibrous, 279

R

Royal College of Physicians of London, 9, 10, 24, 40-41
Royal College of Physicians of Scotland, 17
Royal College of Surgeons, 10, 16
Royal Society of Medicine, 12

S

Scrofula
brain coverings, 263, 269
esophagus, 129
glands, absorbent, 123-124, 164, 168
kidney, 198, 199, 204
larynx, 115
liver, 173-174, 186
lungs, 104
ovary, 252
pericardium, 79, 82
peritoneum, 133-134
pharynx, 121
prostate, 223, 226
seminal vesicles, 220
testicle, 234, 239
trachea, 115, 123
Seminal Vesicles, 220 222
absent (wanting), 221
cul-de-sac, 221
inflammation, 220
scirrhous, 221
scrofula, 220
small, 221
stones, 222
symptoms, 222
Shotts, Lanarkshire, 7
Situs Inversus, 21
Smallpox
intestine, 163
stomach, 144
Soemmerring, Professor, 26, 27, 71
Spermatic Chord, 237-238
edema, 238
sack, 238, 239
scirrhous, 237
symptoms, 239
varicosities, 237
Spleen, 189-194
absence, 193
adhesions, 189
cartilaginous coats, 191
concretions, 192
hard, 190, 194
hydatids, 192, 194
inflammation, 189-190, 193
large, 191-192
mortified, 190
multiple small, 192, 193
rupture, 192
soft, 190
symptoms, 193-194
tubercles, 191
St. George's Hospital, 8, 9, 11
Stomach, 138-145
air distention, 142-145
arsenic, 138-139, 144
calculi, 144
cancer, 140-141, 145
cancer and glands, 141
contracted, 142
dilated, 142
hydrophobia, 139, 145
inflammation, 138-139, 144
papillae, 144
post-mortem, 143
pouch, 141
pustules, 144
pyloric stricture, 141-142
scirrhous, 140-141
smallpox, 144
symptoms, 144-145
tumor
fatty, 143
hairy, 143
ulcers, 139-140, 145
Symptoms, 71-72

T

Testicle, 232-237
abscess, 234
adhesions tunica, 233
blind epididymis, 236

bony, 234
cancer, 234-235
cartilaginous, 235
enlarged, 234
hydatids, 233, 238-239
hydrocele, 232, 238
inflammation, 233-234, 239
scirrhus, 234-235
scrofula, 234, 239
small, 236
stricture vas deferens, 236
symptoms, 238-239
undescended, 236-237
vena mendinensis, 235

Theatre, Anatomic, 8, 9

Thoracic Duct, 123
obstructed, 123
ruptured, 123
varicose, 123

Thyroid, 112-114
bronchocele, 112-113, 126
inflammation, 112, 125
ossification, 114, 126
scirrhous, 113-114, 123, 126
symptoms, 125-127

Thymus, 125
abscesses, 125
calculi, 125
enlarged, 125

Trachea, 115-118
catarrh, 115, 127
croup, 116, 128
inflammation, 115, 127
membranes (polypus), 116-117, 128
ossified rings, 117
scirrhous, 117
scrofula, 115, 123
symptoms, 127-128
tubercles, 117
ulcers, 114, 118, 124

Transactions for the Improvement of Medical and Surgical Knowledge, 19

Tumors
brain, 272, 273, 281
brain coverings, 267, 281
choroid plexus, 278
Fallopian tube, 259
glands, absorbent, cancerous, 164
intestine cancer, 153-154
lungs, 109
mesentery, 165
peritoneum, 134
stomach, 140, 141, 143, 145
testicle, 234-235
uterus, 240, 241-242, 248, 249
vagina, 260-261, 263

Tumor Spread
bone to lung, 109
glands, 124
rectum to bladder, 209
rectum to uterus, 209
stomach to glands, 141
stomach to peritoneum, 134

U

Ulcers
bladder, 208, 218
duodenum, 153
esophagus, 113-140
gallbladder, 181-182, 188
genitalia, external, 265
heart, 83
pharynx, 121
stomach, 139-140, 145
trachea, 114
urethra, 229
vagina, 260, 263

Ureter
abscess, 199
calculi, 202
obstruction, 202

Urethra, 227-231
abscesses, 227
caruncle, 229, 231
Cowper's glands, 228
fistula, 227
hypospadias (preternatural orifice), 230
inflammation, 228-229, 230
obstruction, 224, 225, 227, 229
stone, 227-228
stricture, 229, 230
symptoms, 230-231
ulcers, 229

Uterus, 240-250
bicornuate, 247

bony, 244, 245
contracted os, 244
hydatids, 246-247, 250
inflammation, 240, 248
inversion, 243, 249
leiomyoma (tubercle), 241-242, 249
lithopedion, 245
malignant ulcer, 240, 248
polypus, 242-243
pregnant, 240, 247
prolapse, 244, 249
rupture, 247, 250
scirrhous, 241, 248
stricture, 244
symptoms, 248-250

V

Vagina, 260-263
adhesions, 260, 263
hermaphrodite, 261
inflammation, 260, 262-263
inversion, 261, 263
narrow, 262
polyps, 262
recto-vaginal fistula, 157, 208, 260
short, 262
symptoms, 262-263
tumors, 260-261, 263
ulcers, 260, 263
vagino-vesicular fistula, 260
Varicosities
spermatic cord, 237
vena azygous, 122
Vena Azygous, 122
rupture, 122
varicose, 122
Vena Cava, Inferior
obliterated, 122
Venereal, 265
Vesalius, 17

W

Wardrop, James, 11, 16, 19, 26
Worms, 25, 157-167
Ascaris, 161, 167
Earthworms, 157-159
liver, 178
Lumbricus teres, 157-159, 167
Taenia lata, 160
Taenia solium, 159-160, 167
Trichuris, 161